ANNE HOOPER'S

KAMA
SUTRA

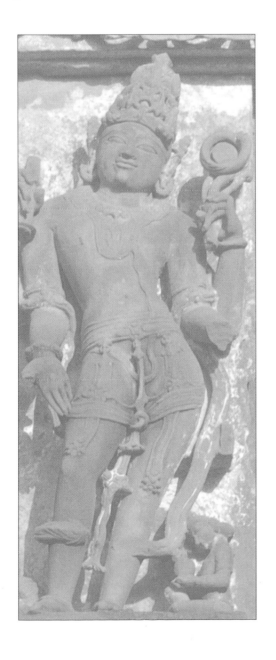

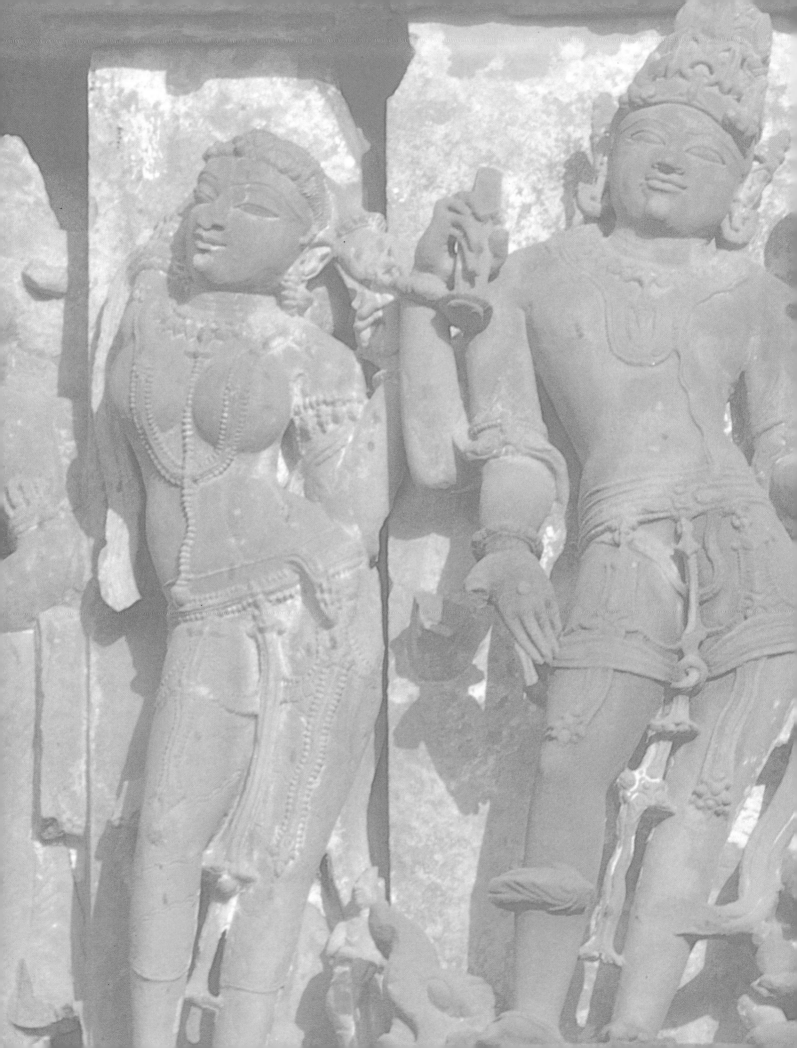

ANNE HOOPER'S
KAMA SUTRA

Classic lovemaking techniques reinterpreted
for today's lovers

A DK PUBLISHING BOOK
www.dk.com

A DK PUBLISHING BOOK
www.dk.com

Created and produced by
CARROLL & BROWN LIMITED
5 Lonsdale Road
London NW6 6RA

Editorial Director Amy Carroll
Project Editor Ian Wood
Contributing Editor Richard Dawes

Design Director Denise Brown
Art Editor Gary Cummins
Designers Carmel O'Neill
Juanita Grout

First American Edition, 1994
8 10 9 7

Published in the United States by
DK Publishing, Inc.
95 Madison Avenue,
New York, NY 10016

Library of Congress Cataloging-in-Publication Data
Hooper, Anne
[Kama Sutra]
Anne Hooper's Kama Sutra . — 1st ed.
p.   cm.
Includes index.
ISBN 1-56458-649-9
1. Sex.   2. Love.   3. Sexual intercourse.   I. Title: Kama Sutra
HQ31.H737   1994
306.7–dc 20
94–21871
CIP

Reproduced by Colourscan, Singapore
Printed and bound in Hong Kong by
Dai Nippon Co., (Hong Kong) Ltd.

CONTENTS

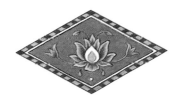

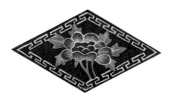

INTRODUCTION

When I was first asked to write a commentary for a new edition of the Kama Sutra, I was less than enthusiastic. In the '60s and '70s there seemed to be dozens of versions

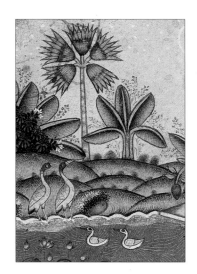

of the Kama Sutra. All were removed from my own lifestyle, and I didn't feel there was much I could relate to in the text. Although I'm fascinated by human sexual nature, I'm not very interested in sex practiced as a style of gymnastics. I would defend freedom for the aficionado of sophisticated sexual positions, but I've never felt that athletic poses had much to do with my own sex life. So it was with reluctance that I sat down and began to read a copy of the Burton and Arbuthnot translation, which was first published in 1883 and which I have quoted extensively in this book. To my surprise, I got far more out of the experience than I'd thought possible. I began to understand the sense of humor behind some of the more exotic poses and realized that many of the poses were not just about sex—they were also about the union of body and mind. Some of the sexual poses in the Kama Sutra are yoga positions, and the goal of yoga is to create mental and physical harmony. The Kama Sutra makes sense in our sophisticated world in that we still strive for the experience of ecstasy.

The *Kama Sutra* and its associated texts, the *Ananga Ranga, The Perfumed Garden,* and the *Tao*, are not as baldly sexual as we might assume. There is a connection between these ancient writings and life in the 20th century. It's a connection that centers on feelings. Although it is possible for us to interact sexually with many people, unless we have also cultivated some love and warmth toward the person who is arousing us, we won't get near the real goal of *kama*. The concept of *kama* involves the "enjoyment of appropriate objects by the five senses of hearing, feeling, seeing, tasting, and smelling, assisted by the mind together with the soul." As a concept, *kama* is just as relevant to us now as it was to the Indians in around AD 400.

The *Kama Sutra* may have been produced at any time between AD 100 and AD 400, and it was written in an India that no longer exists. In those days, the ideal citizen cultivated an ideal life. He surrounded himself with friends, made love as if it were an art form, ate and drank well, was interested in painting and music, and regarded himself as a fair lord and master.

The *Kama Sutra* was written for the nobility of ancient India, by a nobleman. Vatsyayana thought of life as consisting of *dharma*, *artha*, and *kama*. *Dharma* was the acquisition of religious merit; *artha* was the acquisition of wealth; and *kama* was the acquisition of love or sensual pleasure. These ideals are not that dissimilar from the codes we live by today. Although we aren't so focused on religious merit any more, we do pursue self-knowledge and personal growth; most of us would like to

have enough money to enjoy a comfortable lifestyle; and most of us would like to be involved in a loving sexual relationship. The main difference is that the world today is far more egalitarian than it was in the time of Vatsyayana. The *Kama Sutra* was intended as a sort of businessman's textbook—only the subject matter is

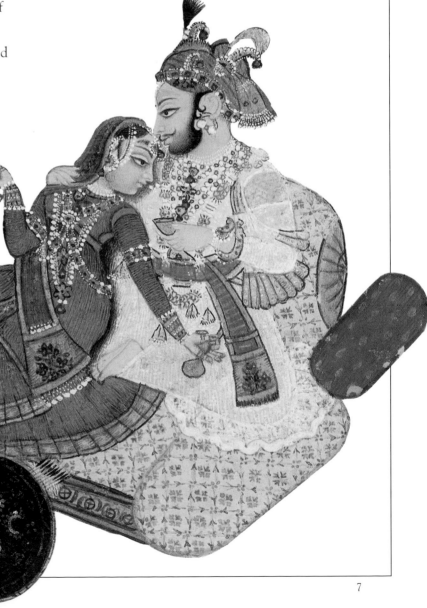

Indian painting,
18th century.

not money, but sex. It was aimed at men because women had very low status then. That isn't to say that women's needs are ignored in the text—they aren't. Pages of detail are aimed purely at exciting the female partner. The instructions concerning female stimulation are explicit. The "work of a man" includes kissing, pressing, stroking, and scratching, and, if a woman should fail to be satisfied by the act of intercourse, Vatsyayana suggests, "the man should rub the yoni [vulva] of the woman with his hand." He even advocates specific sexual positions to suit the sexual match of a couple. "High" congress (*see* The Position of the Wife Of Indra, *page 71*) permits the maximum penetration when a man with a small lingam or linga (penis) makes love to a woman who has a deep vagina. "Low" congress (*see* The

Twining Position, *page 75*) allows easy penetration for a man with a large penis and a woman with a small vagina.

Although the *Kama Sutra* tends to be thought of as a book about sex, it is also a book about manners, conduct, and the arts that a cultivated individual was meant to practice. Although some of the things in the original manuscript would be thought of as peculiar in modern times (the art of teaching parrots and starlings to speak, for instance), there are many sensual arts, such as the use of perfumes, music, and foods, which all translate well into modern sexual practice.

In this version of the *Kama Sutra* I have not only selected the parts of the original text that are still relevant; I have also kept some chunks of 2,000-year-old information because they are in fascinating contrast to the lives we lead today. I have made a point of commenting on aspects of age-old sexual positions, now that we know exactly why we find some of them more stimulating than others. I have also placed special emphasis on the pressure points most likely to give us pleasure. In the past 40 years, we have carried out a great deal of research into human sexuality. Many researchers

Indian painting, late 15th century.

and sexologists, such as Masters and Johnson, Kinsey, and Shere Hite, have documented a wide range of sexual activity, from masturbation to foreplay and intercourse. One of the many tragedies of Hitler's Third Reich was that it resulted in the destruction of decades of sexual research, which American researchers only truly caught up with in the 1970s. On a more personal level, can you imagine anyone in your family handing down the small print of sexual experience from one generation to another? I would be very surprised if your parents told you the intimate details of their own sexual experiences. We don't talk openly about these things. Texts about love and sex, such as the *Kama Sutra*, are few and far between, but they provide us with a valuable historical and cultural perspective on sex.

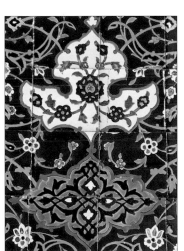

OTHER LOVE TEXTS
I had been pleased and surprised to discover new items of sexual information from reading this ancient text, so I decided to take a look at some of the other early sex manuals.

The *Kama Sutra* was just one of the many Eastern love texts to be translated and printed in the Western world, and for this we must thank the famous Victorian explorer Sir Richard Burton and his colleague Forster Fitzgerald Arbuthnot. The *Ananga Ranga, The Perfumed Garden*, and the *Tao*—which are also featured and quoted in this book—have a lot to offer as well.

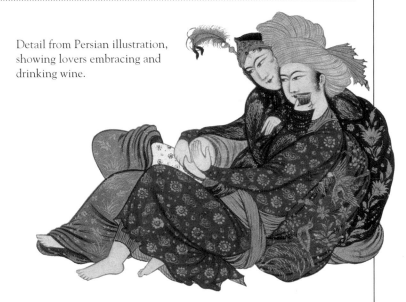

Detail from Persian illustration, showing lovers embracing and drinking wine.

THE ANANGA RANGA
Two years after the publication of the *Kama Sutra* in the West, Burton and Arbuthnot brought out the *Ananga Ranga*. This text was aimed specially at preventing the separation of husband and wife. As the author, Kalyana Malla, says, "The chief reason for the separation between the married couple and the cause, which drives the husband to the embraces of strange women, and the wife to the arms of strange men, is the want of varied pleasures, and the monotony which follows possession." Written around AD 1172, the *Ananga Ranga* is a collection of erotic works, including details from the *Kama Sutra*. Its title translates into "Stage of the Bodiless One," a reference to the story of how Kama, the Hindu god of love, became a bodiless spirit when his physical body was burned to a pile of ashes by a stare from the third eye of the god Shiva.

The book appeared shortly before the start of the Crusades—a time of great cultural exchange between East and West. The returning Crusaders brought many new practices back to Europe with them, including some concerned with sex. The tough warlords of the Crusades who survived the years of fighting had enjoyed the education they subsequently experienced in Arabian, North African, and Syrian harems. Skilled lovemaking was one gain; so, too, were some of the niceties

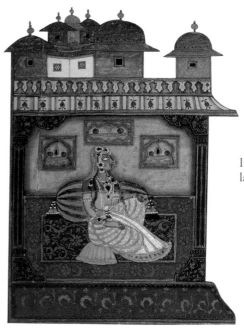

Indian painting,
late 17th century.

of erotic refinement, such as cleanliness and sexual foreplay. It is thanks to these imported Arabian ideas that, in the period after the Crusades, we in the West learned the secrets of how to make love well.

THE PERFUMED GARDEN

It wasn't until Victorian times, however, that any written volume reflecting the ancient and highly imaginative Arabian erotic culture appeared in the West. *The Perfumed Garden* is a translation of an old Arabic manuscript found around the mid-1800s in Algeria by a French officer stationed there. The author of the original manuscript, Sheikh Nefzawi, probably lived in 16th-century Tunis.

When, on later pages, you read some of the details from *The Perfumed Garden*, you will be aware that Sheikh Nefzawi was a man who possessed far greater knowledge of human anatomy and sexual response than did the early Hindus. Perhaps this isn't surprising considering that the Arabs were famed as doctors and could be found at work in many outposts of the Old World. In practical terms, much of Sheikh Nefzawi's advice is well grounded and based on common sense, although it is not always accurate—for example, he recommends that some sexual positions be avoided in that they "predispose for rheumatic pains and sciatica."

Although he may not actually have identified the area we now call the G-spot, he still had a good idea that certain sex positions produced particularly pleasurable sensations in women. It soon becomes clear that Sheikh Nefzawi himself must have been very sexually experienced.

The Perfumed Garden, like the *Kama Sutra*, deals with more than just the mechanics of sex. Sheikh Nefzawi also writes about sensual foods, aphrodisiacs, and the types of men and women he perceives as sexually desirable.

The Perfumed Garden was the third of Sir Richard Burton's publications for the Kama Shastra Society (*shastra* means "scripture" or "doctrines," and the Kama Shastra Society existed to translate rare and important texts concerned with love and sex). The original text of *The Perfumed Garden* includes a large section on homosexual practices, which Burton diligently translated. He had just completed this chapter on homosexuality when he died (on October 20, 1890), and his wife, who was opposed to the project, threw the new translation into the fire.

All was not lost, however, because Burton's colleague, Dr. Grenfell Baker, managed to reproduce much of the material from conversations that he had had with Burton before his death.

THE TAO

The *Tao*, which makes up the last part of this book, is a collection of ancient Chinese wisdom. It predates the previous three books, in that this science of life was developed so early as to precede the traditions of ancient Egypt, India, and Greece. The *Tao* is a wisdom that consists of eight pillars: philosophy, revitalization, balanced diet, "forgotten food" diet, healing art, sexual wisdom, mastery, and success. Taoist sexology promotes the use of sex and sexual energy to improve health, harmonize

relationships, and increase spiritual realization. You can find some *Tao* training programs for increasing your sexual energy in my previous book, *The Ultimate Sex Book*.

Taoist thinkers believe that sexual stimulation should be protracted in order to reach the highest levels of arousal. In the last pages of this volume, I have included a selection of the classic *Tao* sexual positions, so that we can see them in contrast with the others. Many varied sex positions are recommended within the *Tao*, and their purpose is mainly to promote the flow of sexual health and energy. A lot of them differ from the Hindu and Arabic poses, and this reflects differences in the way the Chinese actually viewed sex. Think, for example, about the names of some of the sex positions. There's The Galloping Horse, Butterflies in Flight, Swallows in Love, Silkworm Spinning a Cocoon. These are intensely visual descriptions and it is clear that the ancient Chinese perceived lovemaking as an art form. By understanding this perception, we can begin to feel beautiful about ourselves as sexual people and positive about loving our partners.

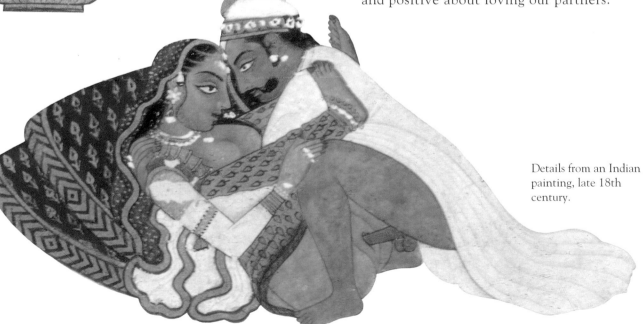

Details from an Indian painting, late 18th century.

USING MY KAMA SUTRA

The original *Kama Sutra* text dealt with a lot more than just sex, but in this book, I have concentrated on the information that relates specifically to sexual foreplay and lovemaking and, where necessary, I have supplemented it with suggestions of my own. For example, I was rather surprised to see that the art of massage wasn't mentioned in the original *Kama Sutra*, and I have included

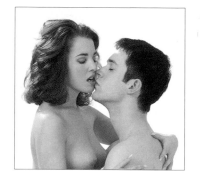

a section on sensual massage *(see pages 34–39)* on the grounds that it is always a wonderful way to begin lovemaking. Moreover, in the final chapter of the book, I discuss another subject that the *Kama Sutra* never tackled: safer sex. Using a condom is an essential part of modern sex, but rather than viewing it as a chore, I have described ways to make it an integral and erotic part of lovemaking *(see pages 154–5)*.

On the pages based on the *Kama Sutra* and other ancient love books, the text set in italics is an interpretation of the original texts, and my accompanying text, set in a plain typeface, is a commentary that aims to place that interpretation in a modern context. Any additional information that I think complements the text is set in boxes.

The first chapter of this book provides an insight into the ancient Indian attitudes about courtship and foreplay, and I have written my own versions of these rituals and the way that we use them today. In the next two chapters, we move on to such details as embracing, mutual grooming, and kissing the lips.

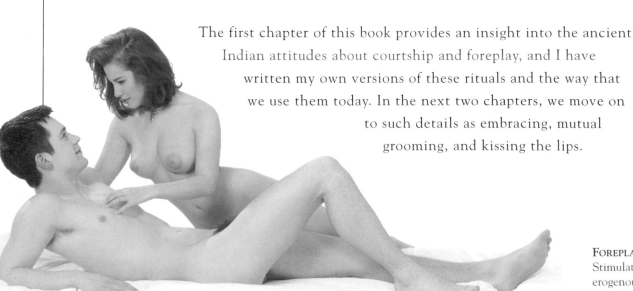

FOREPLAY
Stimulation of the erogenous zones heightens desire.

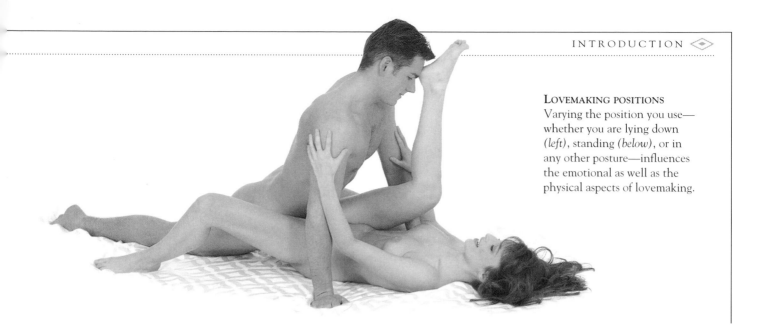

LOVEMAKING POSITIONS
Varying the position you use—
whether you are lying down
(*left*), standing (*below*), or in
any other posture—influences
the emotional as well as the
physical aspects of lovemaking.

Leaving marks on each other's skin is not a practice we endorse
today, yet the idea that pleasure can sometimes be close to
the experience of pain is not so alien to us. Try to keep
an open mind when reading the section on scratching
(*see pages 40–41*). All the practices described in the
Kama Sutra are open to interpretation, and we can
often modify them to meet our own needs.

Who would have thought there are so many different types of kisses? And does it really matter? I think
it does. Different types of kisses have different mean-
ings. Light, sensitive kisses are provocative and can
set the scene for lovemaking; deep tongue kisses can be
as erotic as sex itself. The pages on kissing and mouthplay
(*see pages 46–63*) should help you assess and adapt your
own techniques.

Most of this book is, however, devoted to sex positions
(*see pages 66–149*). Because the *Kama Sutra* offers a
limited choice, I have supplemented those it describes with
positions from other ancient love texts, including the *Ananga
Ranga*, *The Perfumed Garden*, and the *Tao*. If the positions are
very athletic, or seem difficult, I don't hesitate to say so! I just
hope they will inspire you to achieve new heights of ecstasy
with your partner.

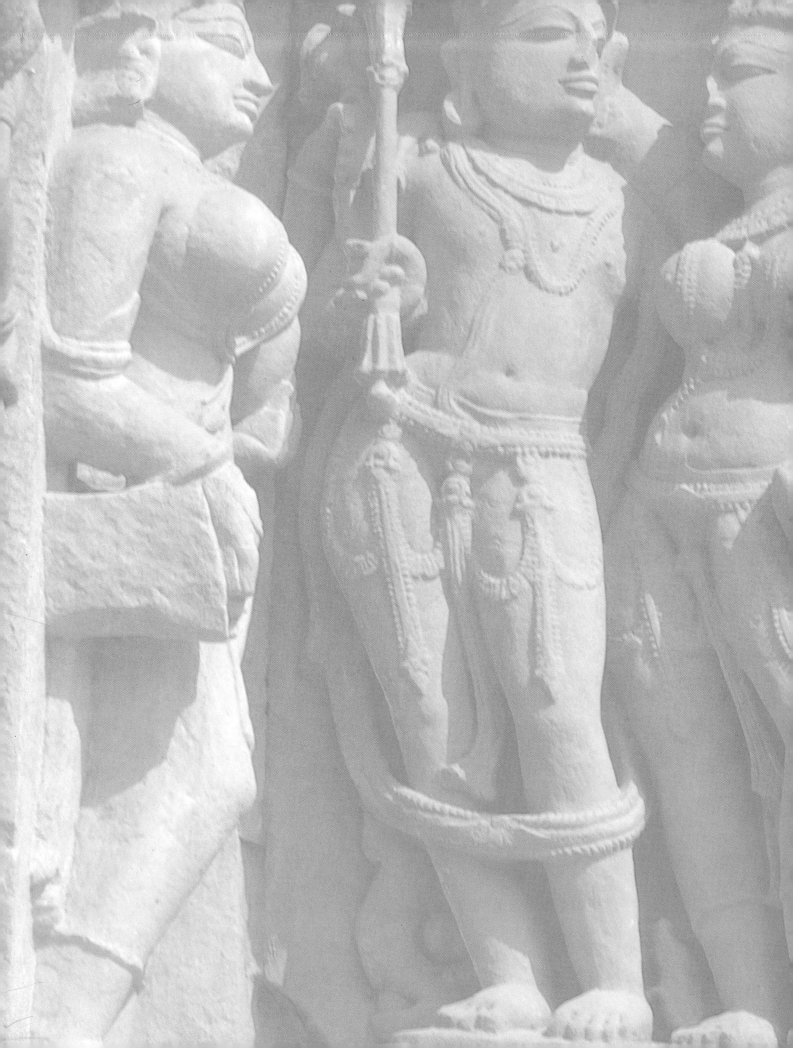

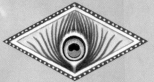

PREPARING
FOR
LOVE

" In all these things connected with love, everybody should act according to his own inclination. "

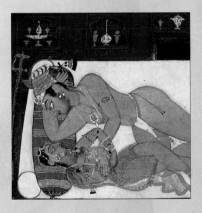

PREPARING THE BODY

In the Hindu tradition that produced the *Kama Sutra*, the human body is seen as a vehicle for expressing spirituality—not, as in the West for many centuries since, as a sinful thing. Sex is celebrated as a sacrament, and the erotic statues and wall carvings seen in Hindu temples throughout India pay testimony to this ancient

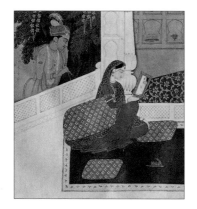

belief. The Hindu tradition regards the body as deserving of being treated with reverence, and in the section describing the "life of a citizen," the *Kama Sutra* details the care it should receive: "Now the householder, having got up in the morning and performed his necessary duties, should wash his teeth, apply a limited quantity of ointments and perfumes to his body, put some ornaments on his person and collyrium [a medicated eye lotion] on his eyelids and below his eyes, color his lips with alacktaka [a dye], and look at himself in the glass. Having then eaten betel leaves, with other things that give fragrance to the mouth, he should perform his usual business. He should bathe daily, anoint his body with oil every other day, apply a lathering substance to his body every three days, get his head (including face) shaved every four days, and the other parts of his body every five or ten days. All these things should be done without fail, and the sweat of the armpits should also be removed."

Cultural preferences change, and the details are not as important as the principle. Two thousand years later, cleanliness remains a priority for nearly all lovers, and for many the use of fragrances enhances lovemaking. Be sure that what you use on your hair and body appeals not just to you but to your partner, too. Whether you are male or female, a fragrance that does not suit you will probably turn your lover off—whereas one that enhances your essence can only make good sex better still.

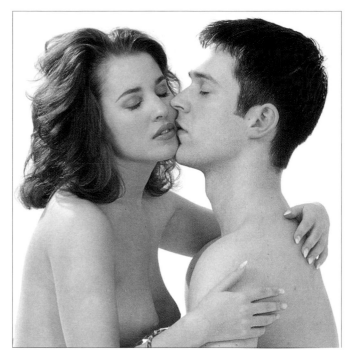

PERFUMING THE BREATH

Body odor alone dampens sexual passion, but when it is combined with bad breath it can kill desire stone dead. Not for nothing does the Kama Sutra recommend remedies for improving the breath. Fortunately, there is a wide range of breath fresheners on the market, and they are probably more effective than the betel leaves suggested by Vatsyayana.

THOSE WHO SUFFER from bad breath are often unaware of the problem—sometimes because their partner does not want to mention it. If you suspect you may be suffering from it, ask your partner to be honest with you. However, when bad breath is serious and constant, the sufferer should seek medical advice rather than simply disguising the problem.

BATHING TOGETHER

Taking a shower together, or sharing the bathtub, not only removes the grime of the day but also gets you in the mood for love. It can be an exciting place to make love (but be careful not to slip), or may be a prelude to bed.

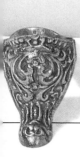

THE EROGENOUS ZONES

It is said that the most potent sexual organ is the brain. The most obvious meaning of this wise dictum is that, without the free play of the imagination, sex can become a soulless and mechanical activity. Male or female, what good lovers have in common is a sensitive and imaginative appreciation of those parts of the body

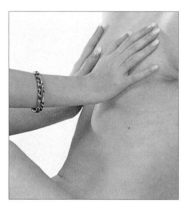

that are rather clinically referred to as the erogenous zones. Perhaps we should call these the pleasure zones, for it is by tapping their erotic potential that you can complement the more extreme joys of which the body is capable. No one who is sexually active would deny that the genitals are one of the primary erogenous zones, along with the brain and the skin. But to concentrate on them to the exclusion of the body's myriad other pleasure zones is like eating part of a well-balanced meal and leaving the rest.

The classic books on Eastern sexual practice share an awareness of the pleasure zones. They speak of these in terms of kissing and touching. Of the kiss, for example, the *Kama Sutra* says that the places where it should be applied include the lips, the inside of the mouth, the forehead, the cheeks, the throat, and the breasts. Most of us also appreciate the potential for pleasure in the nipples, the buttocks, the earlobes, and the feet. The list is as long as you and your partner want it to be. Some people are turned on by having their calves touched, or the inside of their arm. For others, it is anywhere they have skin!

Breasts and nipples
A woman's breasts and nipples are very sensitive, and gentle fondling, squeezing, and kissing can be highly arousing

Lips, neck, and throat
Lightly touching, licking, or kissing these can be spine-tinglingly arousing

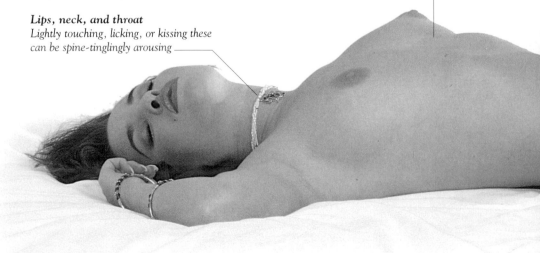

BEST FOOT FORWARD

The feet have reflex connections with the rest of the body, and when stimulated they not only generate pleasurable sensations within themselves but also transmit them all over the body and limbs, and even the head.

IN SOME PEOPLE'S MINDS, the only link between sex and the feet is foot fetishism. However, a clue to the potential of the feet as a source of pleasure lies in their significance in massage and Eastern medicine. The toes are particularly sensitive.

Ankles and calves
Stimulation of some parts of the ankles, calves, and toes can be surprisingly sensual

Thighs
The sensitive inner thighs can be stroked, licked, or kissed for erotic pleasure

Buttocks
These are visually stimulating and richly endowed with nerve endings

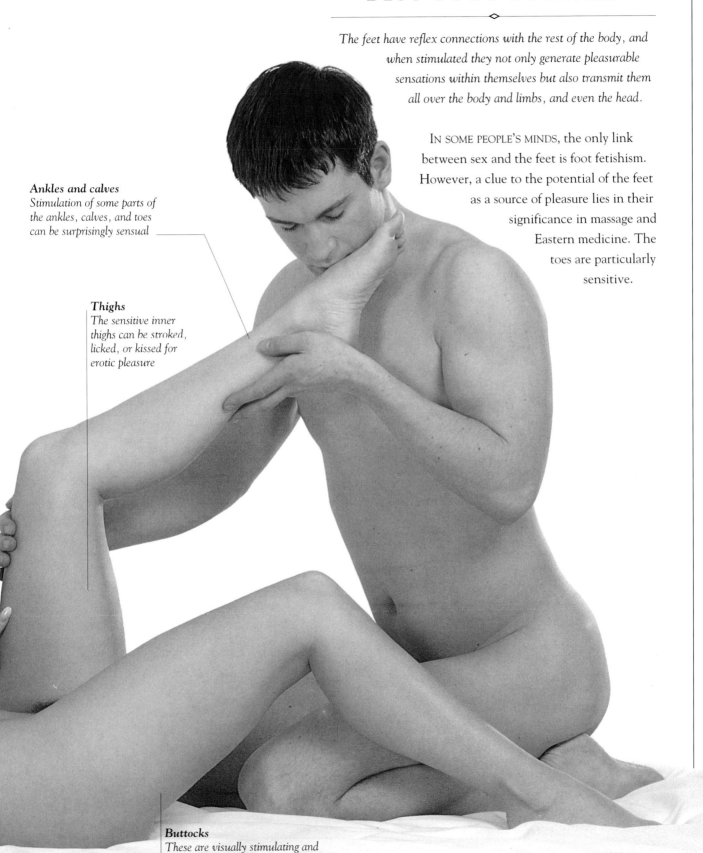

THE SENSUAL SKIN

The skin is the largest organ of the human body, richly endowed with sensitive nerve endings that respond to the lightest touch and the smallest changes in temperature or pressure. For example, on average there are about 1,500 sensory receptors, including touch-sensitive nerve endings, in every square inch of a woman's skin. The skin's sensitivity to stimuli varies from one part of the body to another, and the erogenous zones are among the areas that are especially sensitive to touch.

THE BREASTS

" He should always make a point of pressing those parts of her body on which she turns her eyes. "

A woman's breasts play a major role in sexual attraction. Woman is the only primate female who has swollen mammary glands when she is not producing milk, which highlights the role of the breasts as being more than simply a means of feeding her young. In addition to serving to attract the male, the breasts are undeniably one of the most significant pleasure zones.

THE NIPPLES AND THE surrounding areas (the areolae) are highly sensitive to touch, and some women can reach orgasm by manual or oral stimulation of the nipples alone. Having their nipples rubbed and kissed and their breasts gently squeezed is more important to most women than many men realize. Even those men who are aware that breast stimulation has great potential for giving pleasure often devote less time to the breasts than their partners would like.

Kissing and licking
The nipples are very sensitive, and kissing, licking, and sucking them gently can be highly arousing

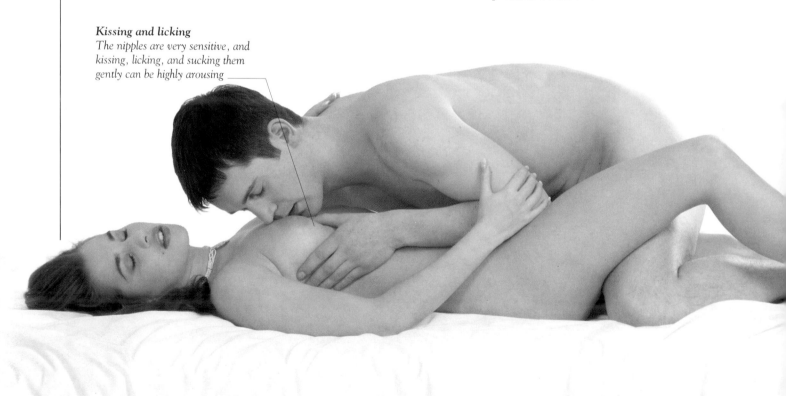

THE BUTTOCKS

Some men find a woman's behind more arousing than her breasts, especially when the buttocks are accentuated by tight clothing. Like the breasts, female buttocks are usually more pronounced than male ones, and with both breasts and buttocks it is their roundness—for most men preferably coupled with firmness—that lies at the heart of their appeal. Although women are less turned on visually than men, some do find the shape of men's buttocks attractive and even sexually arousing. Those who express a preference tend to favor a firm, compact bottom.

LIKE HER BREASTS, a woman's buttocks act both as an attractor, encasing the genitals as they do, and as a source of pleasure. It can be mutually stimulating if the man squeezes, rubs, and lightly slaps them, as well as kissing and biting them gently. The woman may find it enjoyable to do the same for her partner.

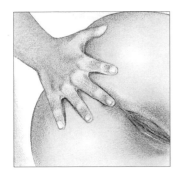

ANAL SENSITIVITY
If you think of a clockface centered on your partner's anus, with 12 o'clock being the point nearest the vagina (or the testicles), the most sensitive and sexually responsive points are at the 10 o'clock and 2 o'clock positions.

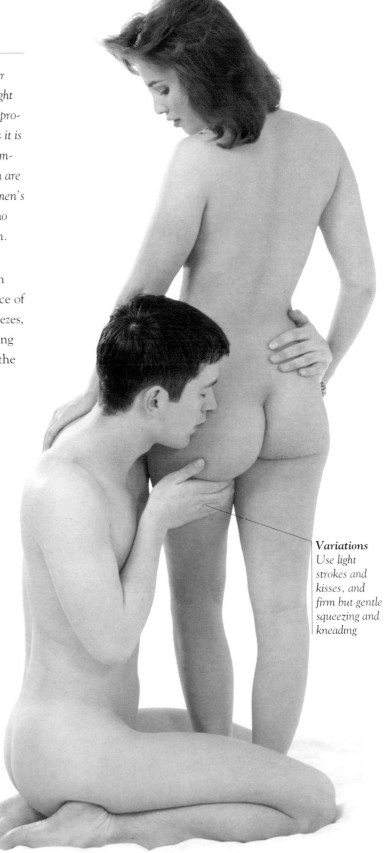

Variations
Use light strokes and kisses, and firm but gentle squeezing and kneading

CREATING THE MOOD

Just as it is important to prepare the body for love, so you should pay careful attention to the room where you and your partner make love. Now, as in the time of the *Kama Sutra*, the way a couple feels about the setting for lovemaking is of prime importance, and in addition to decorating the room with flowers and using fragrances,

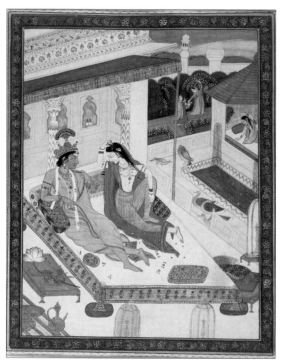

as Vatsyayana suggests, there are a number of other things you can do to create the right atmosphere.

First, make sure that in cold weather the room is warm enough (but not stuffy), and that in hot weather it is refreshingly cool. It is a good idea to provide background music that enhances the mood—neither too raucous or agitated, as this will not be conducive to a tender exchange, nor too soporific, which will make you feel sleepy. Tastes in music vary widely, but it is important to choose something that makes you and your partner feel relaxed and at the same time alert and attentive to each other.

Naturally you will not want to be disturbed, so if you do not have an answering machine, it may be best to unplug the phone or leave it off the hook.

Finally, sexual passion and overindulgence in food and drink may be linked in the popular image of the complete sensualist, but in practice the combination seldom works. While it is often tempting to preface your lovemaking with a lavish meal, or even worse, with a surfeit of alcohol, neither will do anything for you and your part-ner, whether just one or both of you have indulged. Lovemaking is usually best on a satisfied but not overfull stomach, and certainly with a clear head.

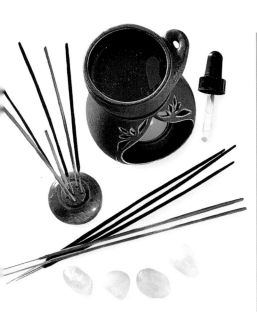

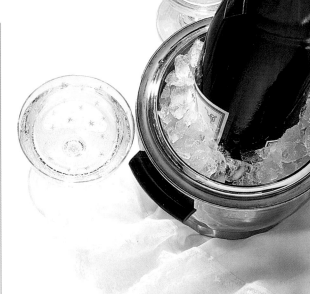

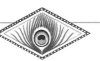

THE SETTING FOR LOVE

Despite the differences between the modern world and the India of the *Kama Sutra*, when we are preparing for lovemaking we would do well to follow the advice of Vatsyayana, who tells us that the room, "balmy with rich perfumes, should contain a bed, soft, agreeable to the sight, covered with a clean white cloth, low in the middle part, having garlands and bunches of flowers upon it, and a canopy above it, and two pillows, one at the top, another at the bottom. There should also be a sort of couch besides, and at the head of this a sort of stool, on which should be placed the fragrant ointments for the night, as well as flowers, pots containing collyrium and other fragrant substances, things used for perfuming the mouth, and the bark of the common citron tree."

SCENTING THE ROOM
Give your bedroom a seductive scent by using incense, heated essential oils, or scented crystals.

PERFUMING THE SKIN
When you bathe, use delicately scented bath oils to perfume and soften your skin. If you prefer a shower to a bath, use a scented shower gel.

FLOWERS
Fresh, fragrant flowers, such as roses, will both decorate and perfume your room.

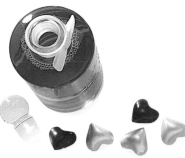

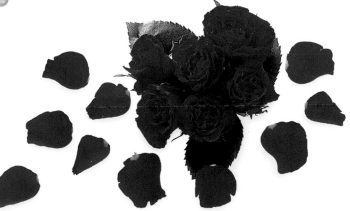

OILS AND LOTIONS
Make your foreplay more seductive by smoothing scented massage oils and lotions into each other's skin. For maximum effect, try giving each other a sensual massage (*see pages 34-39*).

CHAMPAGNE AND SILK
A well-chilled bottle of vintage champagne and seductive silk lingerie or nightwear are two of the traditional ingredients for a romantic evening, whether at home or in a hotel.

SOFT LIGHT
The gentle, flickering glow of candlelight is much more romantic than electric light but, for safety, keep the candles well away from your bedding and other flammable materials. Scented candles will perfume your room as well as casting a soft, seductive light.

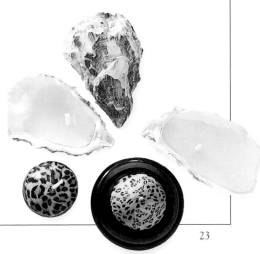

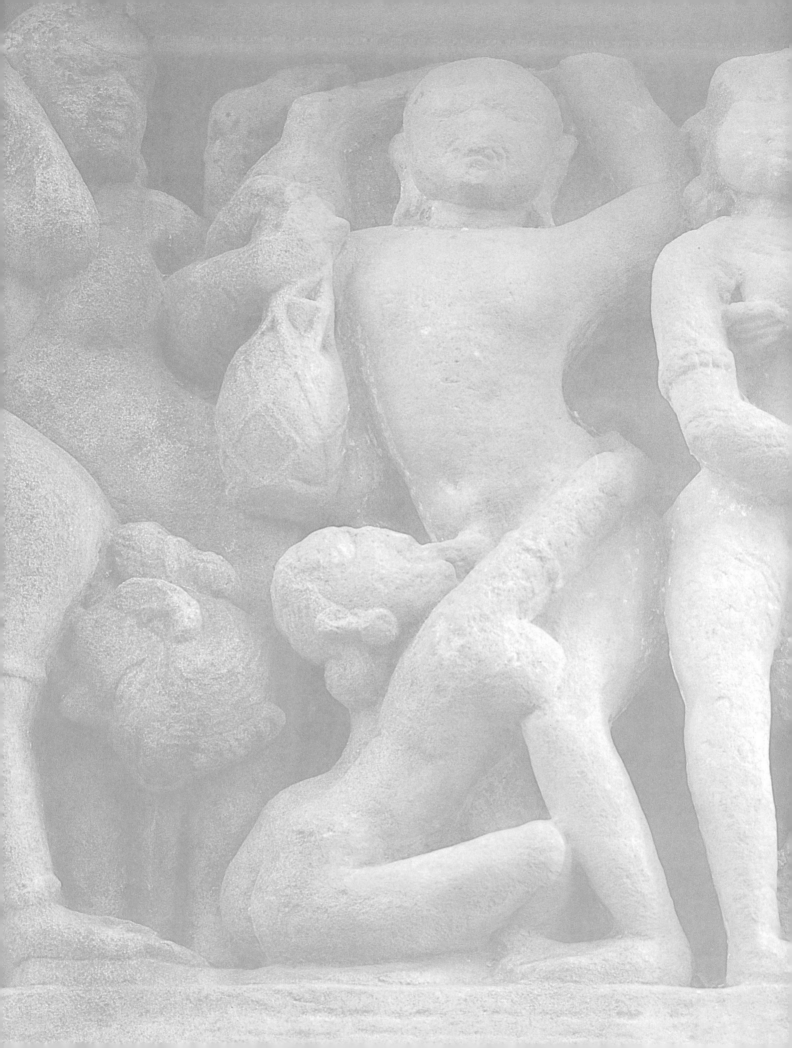

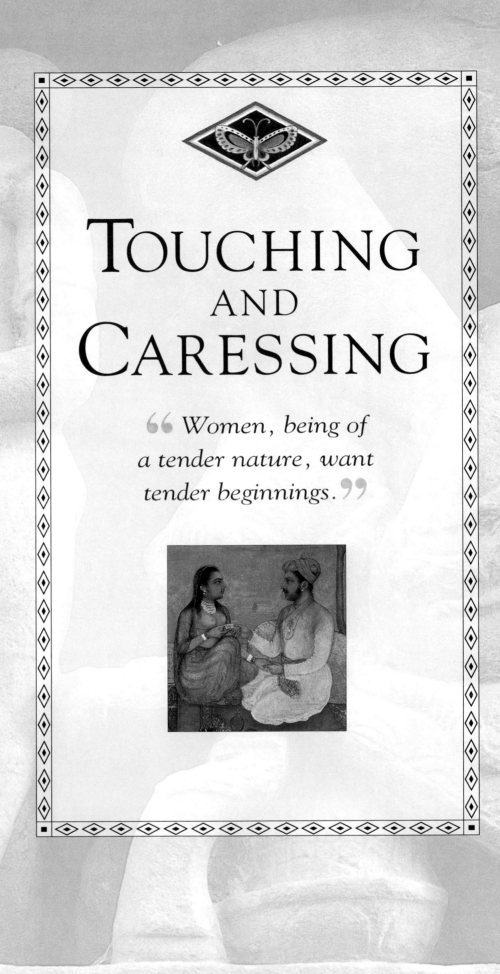

TOUCHING
AND
CARESSING

*“ Women, being of
a tender nature, want
tender beginnings. ”*

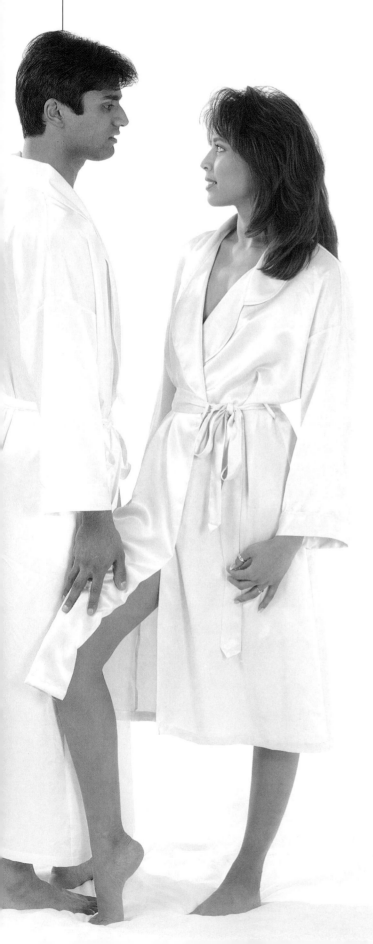

EMBRACING

In discussing the embrace, the *Kama Sutra* begins by dividing it into eight kinds, which form two groups of four. The first group, which "indicate the mutual love of a man and woman who have come together," are the Touching Embrace, the Piercing Embrace, the Rubbing Embrace, and the Pressing Embrace. The second group, embraces that occur "at the time of the meeting," are the Twining of a Creeper (*Jataveshtitaka*), Climbing a Tree (*Vrikshadhirudhaka*), the Mixture of Sesamum [sesame] Seed with Rice (*Tila-Tandulaka*), and the Milk and Water Embrace (*Kshiraniraka*). In addition to these eight embraces, Vatsyayana lists "four ways of embracing simple members of the body"—these "simple members" being the thighs, the *jaghana* (the middle part of the body), the breasts, and the forehead. In describing these embraces, Vatsyayana was probably just categorizing observed behavior rather

THE TOUCHING EMBRACE

The Kama Sutra, *in describing this move, says that "when a man under some pretext or other goes in front of or alongside a woman and touches her body with his own, it is called the touching embrace."*

BETWEEN LOVERS, contrived "accidental" contacts of this type, initiated by either partner, are a playfully erotic way of showing affection.

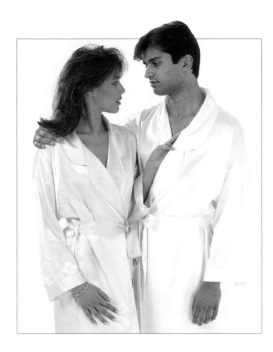

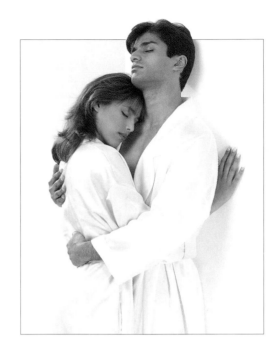

THE RUBBING EMBRACE

"When two lovers are walking slowly together, either in the dark, or in a place of public resort, or in a lonely place, and rub their bodies against each other, it is called a rubbing embrace."

THIS IS A FAMILIAR form of physical contact between lovers, especially younger ones, who when walking together often put an arm tightly around their partner's waist.

THE PRESSING EMBRACE

"When on the above occasion [of the Rubbing Embrace] one of them presses the other's body forcibly against a wall or pillar, it is called a pressing embrace."

MISCHIEVOUSLY LUSTFUL behavior of this sort is, like the Rubbing Embrace, common among young lovers. Being pinned against a wall by a lover is something few people would object to.

THE PIERCING EMBRACE

"When a woman in a lonely place bends down, as if to pick up something, and pierces, as it were, a man sitting or standing, with her breasts, and the man in return takes hold of them, it is called a piercing embrace."

HERE, THE WORD "pierces" is clearly a figure of speech rather than a literal description, and probably means simply that she brushes her breasts against the man as she bends.

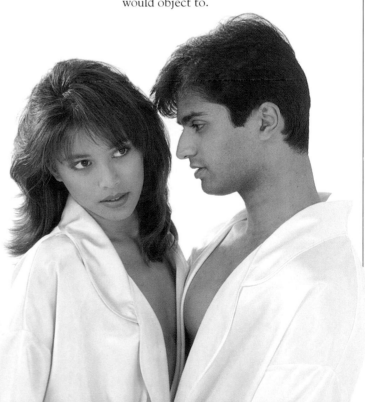

EMBRACING AND LOVEMAKING

Vatsyayana divides the four embraces that are given at "the time of the meeting" into two groups. The Twining of a Creeper and Climbing a Tree are used when the lovers are standing but not in sexual union, while the Mixture of Sesamum Seed with Rice and the Milk and Water Embrace are adopted during congress.

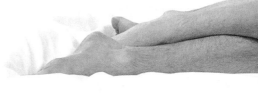

THE MILK AND WATER EMBRACE

"When a man and a woman are very much in love with each other, and, not thinking of any pain or hurt, embrace each other as if they were entering into each other's bodies either while the woman is sitting on the lap of the man, or in front of him, or on a bed, then it is called an embrace like a mixture of milk and water."

THIS EMBRACE has a name evocative of a total mingling, and it graphically describes how lovers try to lose themselves in each other, especially early in their physical relationship.

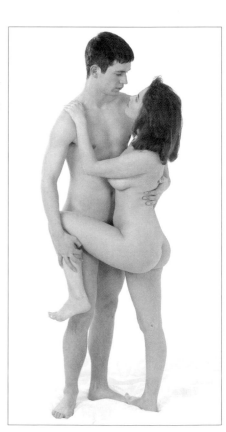

CLIMBING A TREE

"When a woman, having placed one of her feet on the foot of her lover, and the other on one of his thighs, passes one of her arms round his back, and the other on his shoulders, makes slightly the sounds of singing and cooing, and wishes, as it were, to climb up to him in order to have a kiss, it is called an embrace like the climbing of a tree."

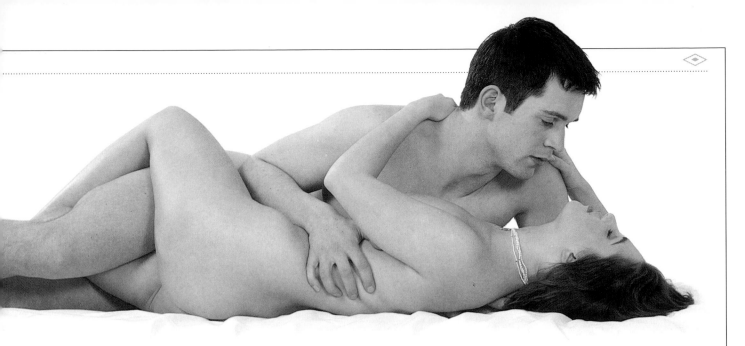

THE MIXTURE OF SESAMUM SEED WITH RICE

◇

"When lovers lie on a bed, and embrace each other so closely that the arms and thighs of the one are encircled by the arms and thighs of the other, and are, as it were, rubbing up against them, this is called an embrace like the mixture of sesamum seed with rice."

THE NAME OF THIS embrace poetically evokes the total intermingling of bodies and limbs, maximizing skin-to-skin contact, that is described here.

THE TWINING OF A CREEPER

◇

The Kama Sutra describes this as "when a woman, clinging to a man as a creeper twines round a tree, bends his head down to hers with the desire of kissing him and slightly makes the sound of sut sut, embraces him, and looks lovingly toward him, it is called an embrace like the twining of a creeper."

FROM THIS DESCRIPTION, it appears that Vatsyayana assumed the woman would be shorter than the man, which was probably as common in his time as it is today. The *sut sut* to which he refers is his way of trying to put inarticulate sounds into words.

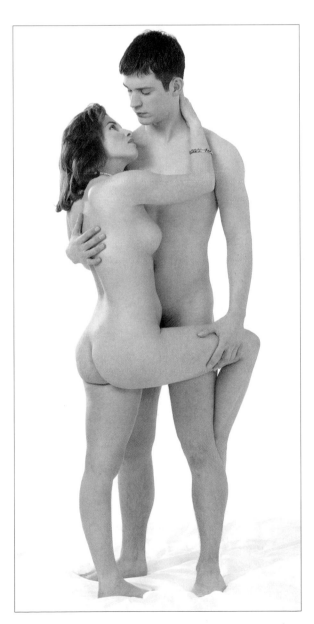

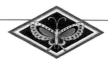

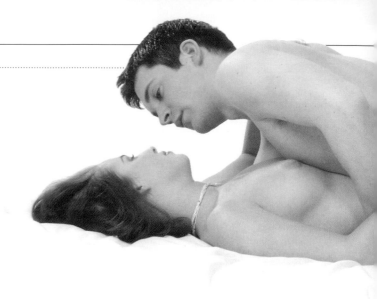

THE AROUSAL OF MALE DESIRE

"The whole subject of embracing," says the *Kama Sutra* (quoting "some verses on the subject"), "is of such a nature that men who ask questions about it, or who hear about it, or who talk about it, acquire thereby a desire for enjoyment. Even those embraces that are not mentioned in the Kama Shastra [the Holy Writ of Kama] should be practiced at the time of sexual enjoyment, if they are in any way conducive to the increase of love or passion. The rules of the Shastra apply so long as the passion of man is middling, but when the wheel of love is set in motion, then there is no motion and no order."

THE EMBRACE OF THE JAGHANA

"When a man presses the jaghana, or middle part of the woman's body, against his own, and mounts upon her to practice, either scratching with the nail or finger, or biting, or striking, or kissing, the hair of the woman being loose and flowing, it is called the embrace of the jaghana."

THE WORD *jaghana* is the term the *Kama Sutra* uses to describe the area between the navel and the thighs. This embrace is clear prelude to intercourse, but most lovers today would dispense of the ritualized scratching, biting, and striking that Vatsyayana recommends.

THE EMBRACE OF THE THIGHS

"When one of two lovers presses forcibly one or both of the thighs of the other between his or her own, it is called the embrace of the thighs."

IN ADDITION TO BRINGING the thighs together intimately, this move can also bring the lovers into contact with each other's genitals, helping to increase arousal and desire.

Full arousal
From this position, lovers move naturally on to intercourse once both are fully aroused

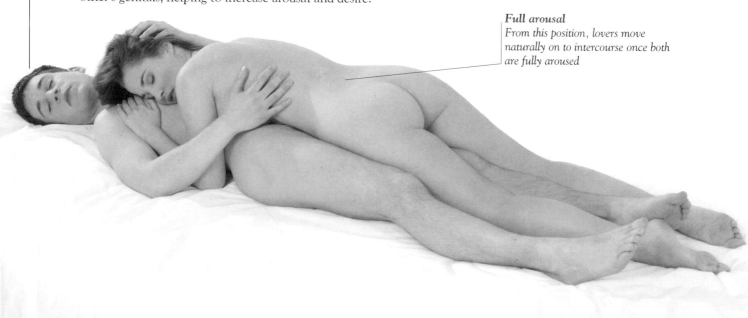

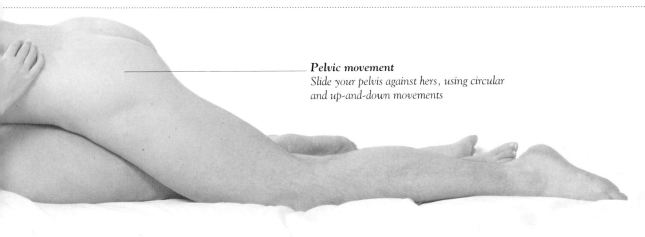

Pelvic movement
*Slide your pelvis against hers, using circular
and up-and-down movements*

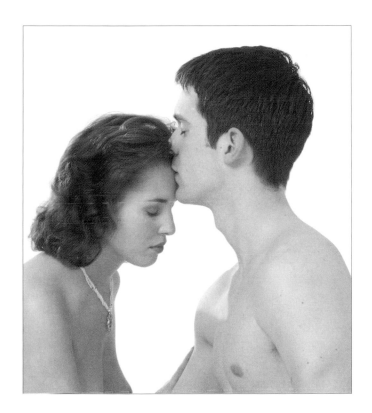

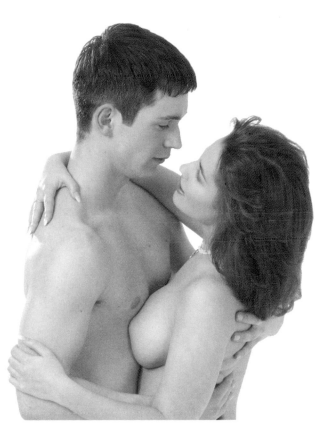

THE EMBRACE OF THE FOREHEAD

*"When either of the lovers touches the mouth, the eyes, and the
forehead of the other with his or her own, it is called the embrace
of the forehead."*

AFFECTIONATE NUZZLING, especially when combined with
kissing, is a useful way to foster intimacy and confidence as
well as to enhance arousal.

THE EMBRACE OF THE BREASTS

*"When a man places his breast between the breasts of a
woman and presses her with it, it is called the embrace
of the breasts."*

UPPER-BODY CONTACT like this provides both partners with
nipple stimulation, and makes an interesting change from
the more usual manual or oral caresses.

MUTUAL GROOMING

Although the *Kama Sutra* indicates that bodily cleanliness should not be overlooked by lovers, it says nothing of mutual grooming. Cultural differences probably account for what many today would regard as an omission: lovers can enjoy a great deal of shared pleasure in preparing for lovemaking. This preparation can include taking a bath or shower together, shaving the man's face, and washing, drying, and brushing each other's hair. Mutual grooming is by no means an indispensable ritual, but by delaying the consummation of love, and focusing the couple's attention on each other's attractions, it can heighten the anticipation of pleasure. It also encourages feelings of tenderness, trust, and caring, enabling each partner to feel protective toward the other. This can help break down inhibitions in a new relationship, and will reinforce the bonds of an established one.

SHAVING HIS BEARD

The Kama Sutra, *surprisingly, recommends that a man shave no more often than every four days. But today, even if a woman thinks a few days' stubble makes her partner look more rugged, she will most likely prefer not to be grazed by his growth when he kisses her. As an alternative to asking him to shave before making love, she could try shaving him herself.*

SHAVING IS NOT JUST for men, because many women shave their legs and armpits and some shave off their pubic hair; some people find a hairless pudendum very erotic. If a woman shaves her pubic hair, she will need to shave it regularly, because new growth will soon be strong enough to irritate her partner's skin.

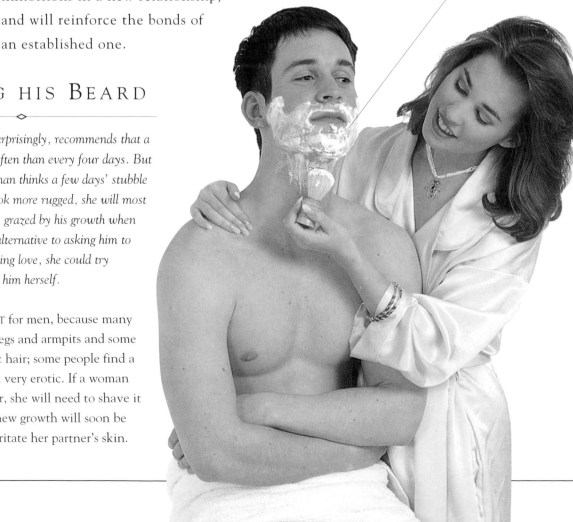

Lather well
Apply a generous layer of foam to ensure a smooth shave with no cuts

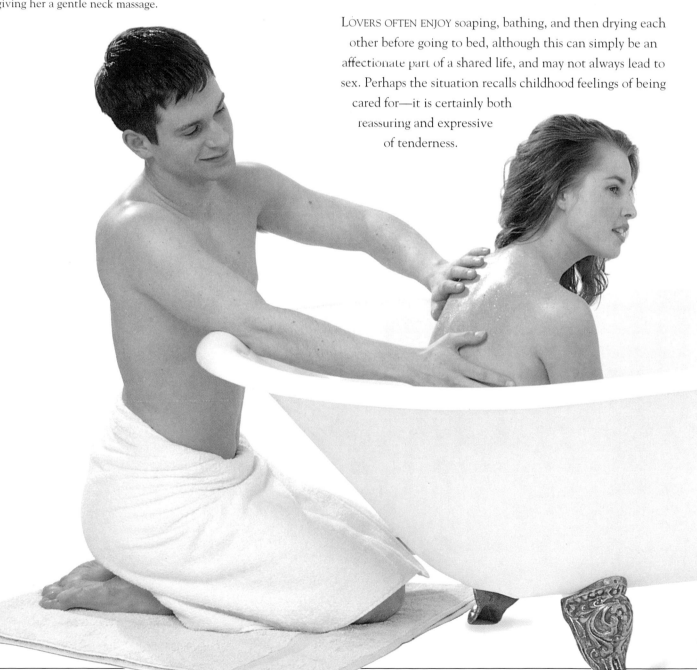

NECK MASSAGE
Before shampooing your lover's hair, help her relax by
giving her a gentle neck massage.

SHAMPOOING HER HAIR

*Vatsyayana says that some people see shampooing as a form of
embrace, but he disagrees with this view because shampooing is
not performed during lovemaking, nor is it done for the same
reasons as an embrace. As a prelude to a lovemaking session,
however, it is a sensuous form of mutual grooming. Whether it is
the hair that is washed or, as in the original meaning of the word
"shampoo," the body is washed and massaged, it can be a very
intimate experience when shared.*

LOVERS OFTEN ENJOY soaping, bathing, and then drying each
other before going to bed, although this can simply be an
affectionate part of a shared life, and may not always lead to
sex. Perhaps the situation recalls childhood feelings of being
cared for—it is certainly both
reassuring and expressive
of tenderness.

SENSUAL MASSAGE

Massage is not described in the *Kama Sutra*, but for thousands of years it has been valued as a means of soothing away tiredness and tension. And yet, because we link touch with sex, we tend to steer clear of touching each other for fear of being misunderstood. This habit can even extend, inappropriately, to our partners, so that we concentrate on purely sexual expression, avoiding any systematic sensual touching. By ignoring the power of massage, many lovers miss out on a source of great pleasure as well as a means of making the body much more receptive and relaxed for lovemaking.

Whether or not it is intended as a prelude to making love, the aim of sensual massage is maximum relaxation, and so it is important to create a peaceful and comfortable setting. A large bed with a firm mattress, or even a sheet on the floor, will be suitable. Place pillows or cushions under your partner's neck, small of the back, and ankles. Make sure that the room is warm and softly lit, and try to ensure that you will not be interrupted. You can use these massage moves individually, combine two or more of them, or build them all into a full sequence, starting at the feet and working up to the head.

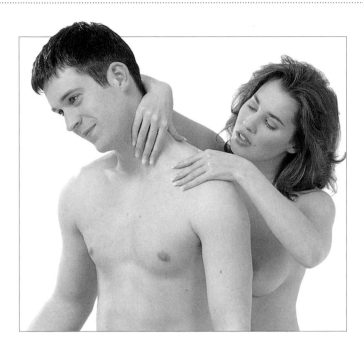

SHOULDERS AND HEAD

Massage the front of the shoulders, the sides of the neck, the cheeks and the jaw, and then the temples and forehead. Run your fingers lightly over the chin and around and over the lips, eyes, and nose, all of which by now should be pleasantly sensitized. Many people also like to have the top of the head massaged, with an action similar to that used in washing hair.

BACK AND SPINE

When massaging the back, use gentle, erotic pressure and work upward from the buttocks, keeping your hands outspread and level with each other and your thumbs pushing inward along the spine. Work up to the base of the neck and then out to the shoulders before bringing your hands slowly down the sides to the buttocks. Repeat this massage about ten times, or more if your partner wishes it.

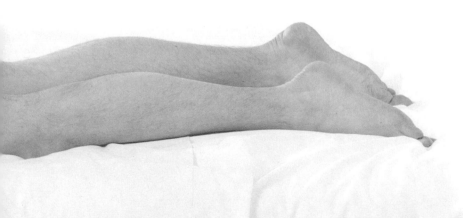

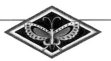

THE BASIC MASSAGE STROKES

You can learn the essentials of massage fairly quickly, and all of the following actions are recommended.

EFFLEURAGE
Glide your palms across the skin, putting your body weight behind the movement. This action should be used first and last on each area.

KNEADING
With your hands gently curved, knead the flesh with a smooth, regular movement.

PÉTRISSAGE
Move the balls of your fingers or thumbs in a circular motion to soothe away any muscular tension along the spine. Do not, however, massage the spine itself.

HACKING
Giving a series of brisk chops with the side of the hand, as in karate but gentler, is known as hacking. Keep your fingers relaxed rather than stiff.

TAPOTEMENT AND CUPPING
Tapotement involves drumming with a light tapping action. Cupping is pounding the body with alternate hands that are cupped with fingers together and thumbs folded in.

Whichever massage technique or stroke you use, always keep your movements even, rhythmic, and symmetrical, and follow each one through where appropriate. Always use a suitable oil *(see page 37)*, and agree with your partner on the amount of pressure to be used, since this should always be a matter of pleasure for you both. Also, you should learn to forgo your own needs temporarily and concentrate instead on your partner's enjoyment. By doing so, you will attain the prized goal of being able to give and receive pleasure fully.

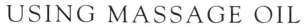

USING MASSAGE OIL

All massage oils work best when they have been prewarmed by rubbing them for a few seconds between the hands. Used cold, they come as a shock to the skin. Oil each area before you attend to it rather than oiling the whole body first: apply a small amount to the part you intend to massage, and rub it into the skin with smooth but firm strokes. After the massage, the oil can be left to soak into the skin. Alternatively, it can be removed by wiping gently with a towel or, more effectively, with rubbing alcohol, although as this must be used cold it can break the spell.

Support
Hold her leg steady with one hand while you massage it with the other

Sit close
To avoid back strain, sit close to your partner so you do not have to bend or stretch forward

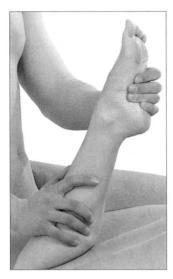

DOWNWARD LEG STROKES
Draw your hand smoothly down
from ankle to knee, and squeeze
the calf muscles gently with
your fingertips.

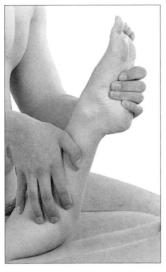

UPWARD LEG STROKES
Using the same sort of action as
when making a downward
stroke, draw your hand back up
the leg from knee to ankle.

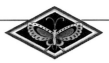

MASSAGE OILS
AND ADDITIVES

You can massage your partner with
dry hands, but your movements will
be smoother, especially if you are
new to it, if you use a massage oil or
an oil-free massage lotion. There is a
wide variety of suitable oils, many
derived from nuts (particularly
coconut) or vegetables. Plain oils
such as almond, olive, grapeseed,
and sunflower can be applied
straight to the skin, or used as bases
for perfumed essential oils such as
patchouli, sandalwood, ylang-ylang,
jasmine, and rose. Make up enough
scented oil for one session by adding
up to a dozen drops of essential oil to
1 fl oz (30 ml) of base oil.

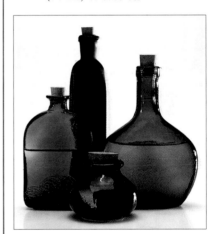

Bottles of massage oil

FEET AND LEGS

◇

With your partner lying facedown, start by massaging the toes—stretching, kneading,
and bending each one upward—before softly rubbing the areas between them. Next, run
the palms of your hands firmly over the soles of the feet and then along the tops. Raise
each leg in turn and gently rotate each foot a few times until it feels loose and relaxed.
Gradually move up the leg, paying special attention to the ankles, calves, and backs of
the knees and the thighs.

Position
Massaging your partner's calves,
ankles, and feet is easier if she
lies facedown

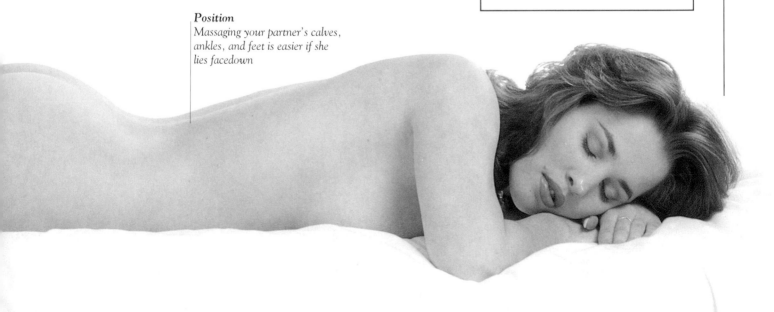

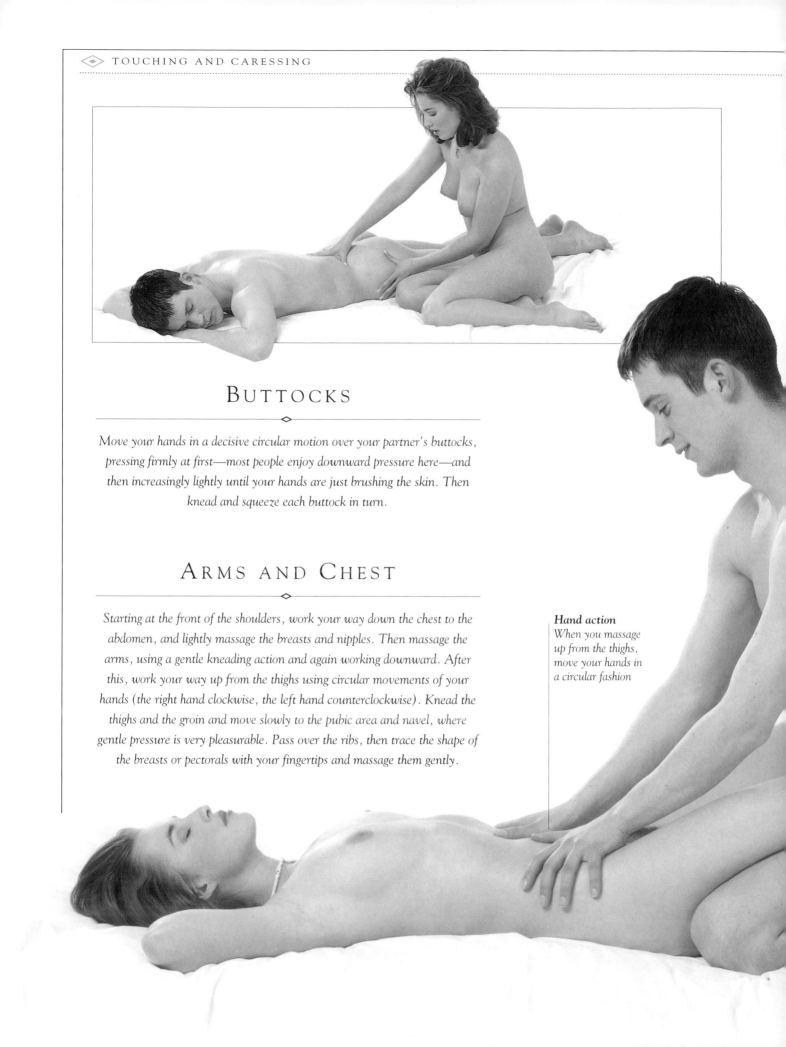

BUTTOCKS

◇

Move your hands in a decisive circular motion over your partner's buttocks, pressing firmly at first—most people enjoy downward pressure here—and then increasingly lightly until your hands are just brushing the skin. Then knead and squeeze each buttock in turn.

ARMS AND CHEST

◇

Starting at the front of the shoulders, work your way down the chest to the abdomen, and lightly massage the breasts and nipples. Then massage the arms, using a gentle kneading action and again working downward. After this, work your way up from the thighs using circular movements of your hands (the right hand clockwise, the left hand counterclockwise). Knead the thighs and the groin and move slowly to the pubic area and navel, where gentle pressure is very pleasurable. Pass over the ribs, then trace the shape of the breasts or pectorals with your fingertips and massage them gently.

Hand action
When you massage up from the thighs, move your hands in a circular fashion

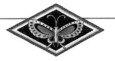

MASSAGE FOR SEXUAL AROUSAL

You can make love better when your body is loosened up by a massage, but if you want to use massage to arouse, rather than just to relax each other, switch from the more vigorous techniques to very gentle actions. For example, tracing a line with the fingertips back and forth across the nipples and chest, or the lower abdomen, can be far more exciting than the more forceful movements of conventional massage.

Many other areas respond to an insistent, "feathering" touch; these include the earlobes, the sides and nape of the neck, the insides of the arms and thighs, the navel, the buttocks, the calves, and the toes. You need not restrict yourself to using your hands: lie on your partner and rub your body against his or hers, or use your feet and toes to explore hidden crevices and provide each of you with novel sensations. If the right chemistry exists between a couple, almost every area of the body is highly sensitive to the erotic touch of the lover and can be stimulated so as to give pleasure and heighten anticipation.

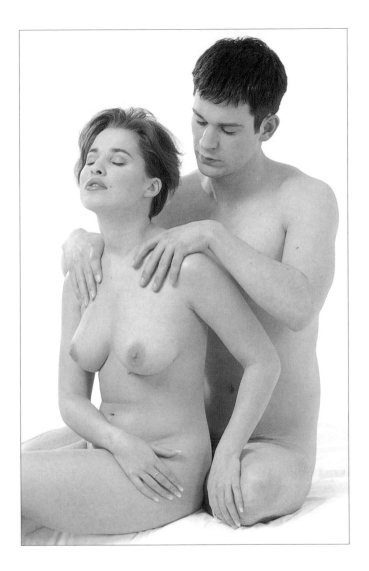

THE UPPER BACK

When you massage the upper back, work on the muscles between the shoulder blades and at the base of the neck. Then bring your hands back down, massaging your partner's sides with your fingertips. Knead the shoulders and, reducing the pressure, the back of the neck.

SCRATCHING

While acknowledging that lovers often use their fingernails to express passion on parting or meeting, or on reconciliation after a quarrel, the *Kama Sutra* says that pressing and scratching with them during lovemaking are techniques restricted to those who find them pleasurable. In the India of the *Kama Sutra*, as in other cultures before and since, marks of passion on a young woman's breast or throat served to tell the world that she was spoken for.

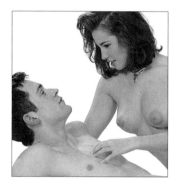

Such marks excite admiration, Vatsyayana explains, so that "even when a stranger sees at a distance a young woman with the marks of nails on her breast, he is filled with love and respect for her." The same goes for a man bearing nail marks. Marks are also exchanged, says the *Kama Sutra*, to remind lovers of each other when they are apart: "If there be no marks of nails to remind a person of the passages of love, then love is lessened in the same way as when no union takes place for a long time." Wives, however, should not be seen bearing such mementoes of love, although it is acceptable for a married woman to have them on her private parts. "In short," Vatsyayana concludes, "nothing tends to increase love so much as the effects of marking with the nails and biting."

Nail pressure
Press hard enough to leave marks but not so hard as to break the skin ⸺

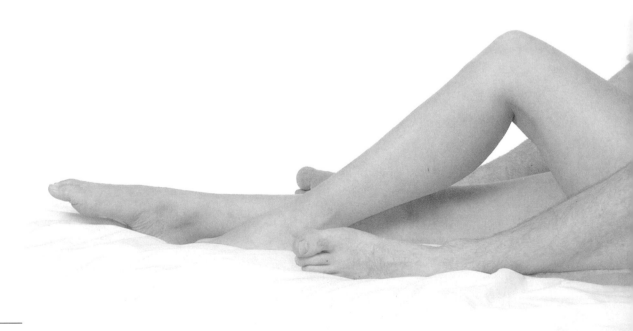

SCRATCHING

While it does not suggest that using the fingernails is to everyone's taste, it is clear that the Kama Sutra regards them as a useful weapon in a lover's armory.

IF LEAVING love marks is based on passion rather than anger or cruelty, both partners may find it fun from time to time.

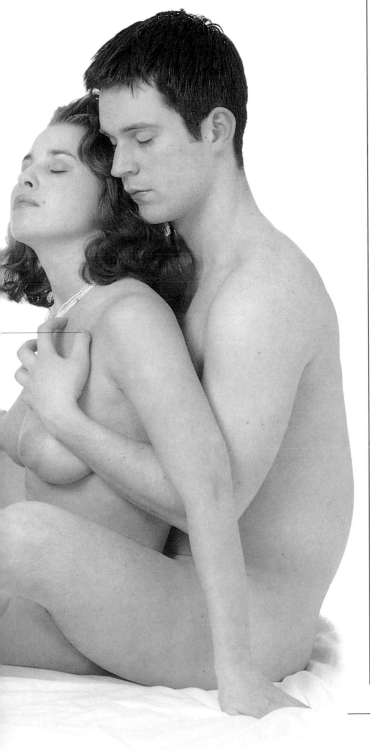

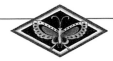

THE RITUALIZED BLOWS OF LOVE

The *Kama Sutra* discusses various ways in which harmless ritual striking can be used by both partners to express their feelings and heighten excitement before and during intercourse. Four kinds of blows are described, using the back of the hand; the fingers, slightly contracted; the fist; and the palm of the hand. The blows are most effective on the shoulders, the head, the space between the breasts, the back, the midriff, and on the sides.

Modern lovers might well use light blows on each other spontaneously, but violence is a very taboo subject in our society—people are afraid of it, and with good reason. And although the Kama Sutra *suggests that the woman should return the man's blows, many* women are frightened and repulsed by such behavior. Those who enjoy ritualized violence are stigmatized in our society, as well as being the butt of many jokes. But the aficionados of spanking, for example, will tell you that a light spank, with the flat of the hand, doesn't actually hurt. It provides a brief, arousing tingling sensation, and if you get enough of these light spanks, your body becomes very aroused. There is an emotional dimension, too. Because the act of striking someone, however ritually, is an aggressive one, many people find that artificial aggressive act can be provocative enough to engage the emotions, to annoy you so that you retaliate and thus bring about a mock fight. This raises your adrenaline levels, and when these are heightened you become turned on.

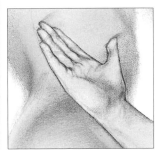

With the back of the hand

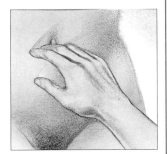

With the fingers

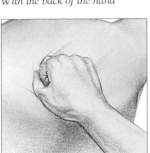

With the fist

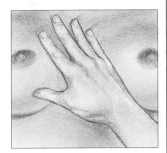

With the palm of the hand

HAIR PLAY

The *Kama Sutra* acknowledges the eternal fascination that a woman's hair has for a man, stating that among the arts she should learn is that of "dressing the hair with unguents and perfumes and braiding it." The power that her hair exerts is reciprocated when, by praising and fondling it, her partner arouses feelings of desire in her, which he then undertakes to satisfy. In Vatsyayana's time, long hair would have graced women and men alike. Now as then, it is a valuable asset in love play. Pubic hair can also feature in the preliminaries to lovemaking, and for lovers, the sight and feel of each other's pubic hair heralds the imminent joys of intercourse. But fondling the pubic hair need not be confined to foreplay, for after lovemaking it can reciprocate tenderness just as eloquently as it can signal the desire to make love again. It should be touched gently—the hairs being stroked rather than pulled.

A LIGHT TOUCH

When it is long, a woman's hair falls beguilingly over her face or breasts and brushes sensually against her partner's naked body. If it is long enough, she can even enfold his shoulders and chest with it. And if she is on top, she can position herself so as to sweep it teasingly over his whole body, including his penis, so heightening his desire for her.

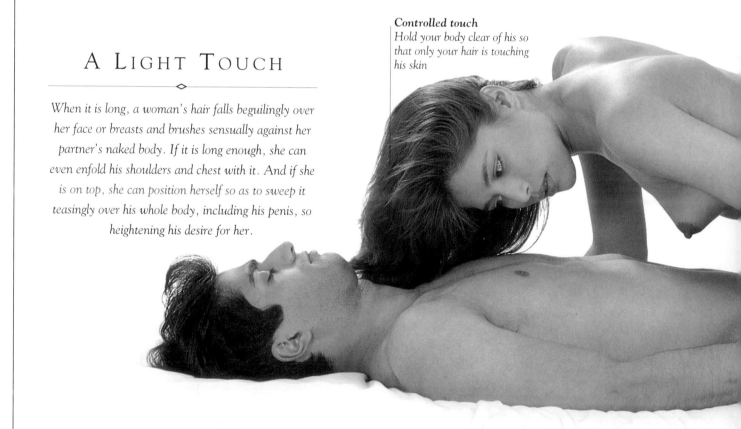

Controlled touch
Hold your body clear of his so that only your hair is touching his skin

REVEALING THE NECK

Clean, lustrous hair can be a powerful aphrodisiac, inviting lovers to toy with it and bury their hands in it. Its texture and sheen are attractive in themselves, but when the hair is lifted to reveal a soft, delicate neck, the joy is even greater.

SOMETIMES A MAN will choose this way to make his desire known to a woman, and the animal connotations of an approach from behind usually provide additional excitement for both partners.

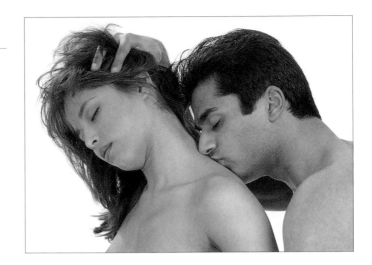

TACTILE PLEASURE

Loving touch is one of the most important parts of an intimate relationship, and by running her fingers through her partner's hair while he plays with hers, a woman can increase the tactile pleasure for both of them.

LOVERS CAN TAKE this a step further by brushing each other's hair or by giving each other a gentle scalp massage.

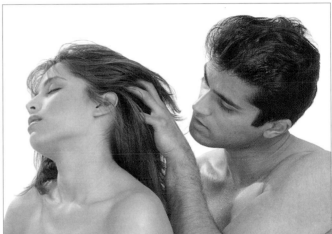

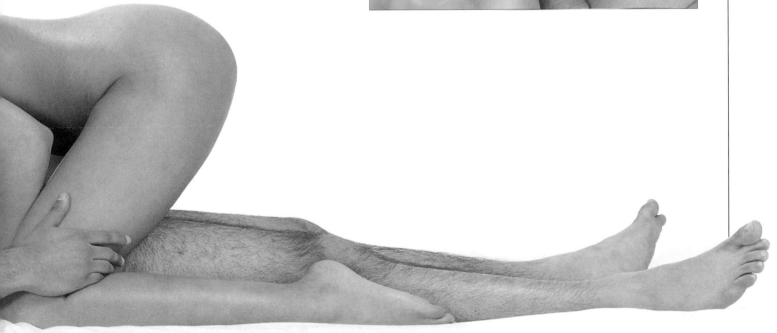

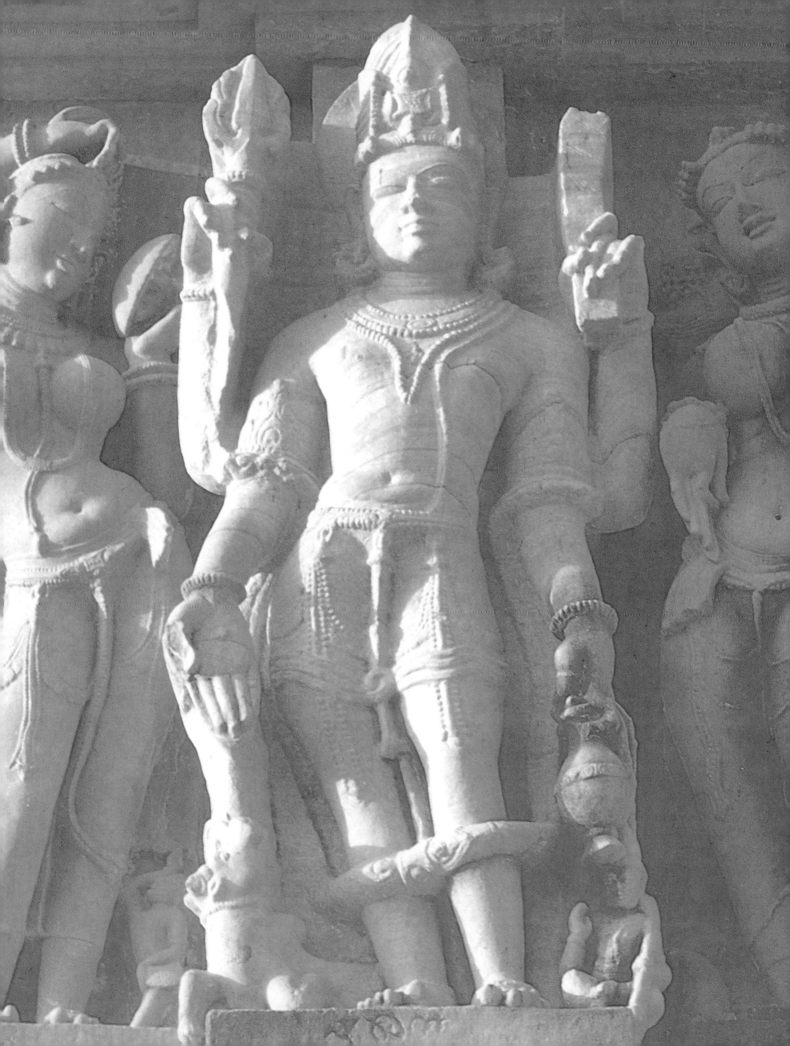

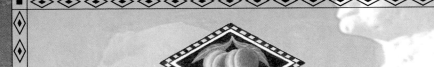

KISSING
AND
MOUTHPLAY

❝ Men and women, being of the same nature, feel the same kind of pleasure. ❞

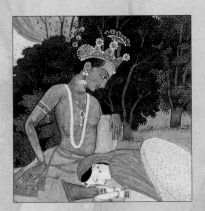

KISSING

The mouth is among the most sensitive parts of the body, and the most versatile—you can use your lips or tongue to kiss, lick, suck, nuzzle, or nibble any area of your partner's body. Kissing is an art in itself, and the *Kama Sutra* recognizes its power of expression by describing in detail the different forms of kissing and when each type of kiss is appropriate. Whatever its intensity, a kiss on the lips combines the three senses of touch, taste, and smell, each of which can produce a strong emotional response. Kisses range from fleeting contact to a deep penetration with the tongue, when the rhythm of the penetration can be matched to that of simultaneous intercourse. In between lie many variations, and perhaps the *Kama Sutra* describes types of kisses in great detail because the skill was as often overlooked then as it is now.

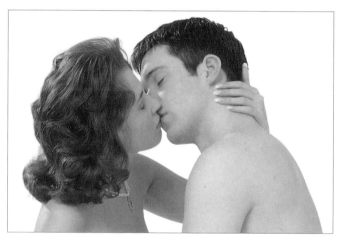

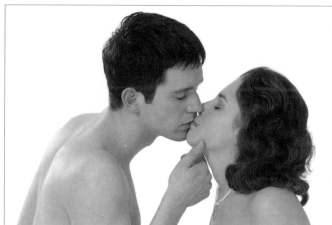

THE BENT KISS

The Kama Sutra's Bent Kiss is what occurs when "the heads of two lovers are bent toward each other, and when so bent, kissing takes place."

ONE OF THE MOST NATURAL ways to kiss your lover is with your head angled slightly to one side, which permits maximum lip contact and deep tongue penetration. It's a superb means of expressing passion during foreplay and a great way to heighten the excitement of intercourse.

THE TURNED KISS

"When one of them turns up the face of the other by holding the head and chin, and then kissing," says the Kama Sutra, *"it is called a turned kiss."*

GENTLENESS AND LOVING tenderness are the principal emotions evoked by a kiss of this type, which is a good one to use at the beginning of foreplay or when you are making love very slowly in a face-to-face sitting or standing position.

THE STRAIGHT KISS

◇

This is the name that the Kama Sutra gives to a kiss in which "the lips of two lovers are brought into direct contact with each other."

WHEN LOVERS KISS like this, with their heads angled only slightly to each side, tongue penetration is impractical. Because of this, the straight kiss is not a means of expressing intense passion, but it is a gentle way of showing affection and expressing the initial stages of desire. It's the kind of kiss that new lovers often use in the earliest, most tentative moments of their physical relationship.

Use your hands
When kissing, use your hands to caress, stroke, and fondle your lover's body

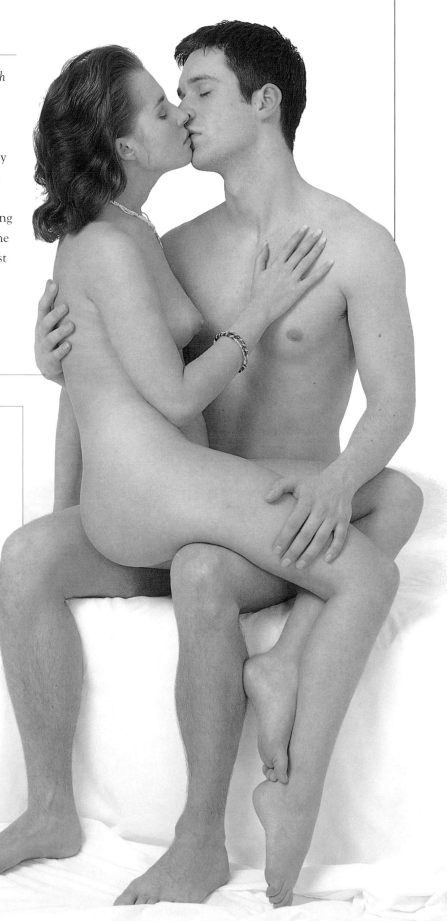

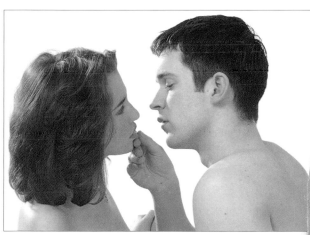

THE PRESSED KISS

◇

There are two versions of this kiss, the first being when "the lower lip is pressed with much force." The second, shown here, is "the greatly pressed kiss," in which one of the lovers holds the other's lower lip and then, after touching it with the tongue, kisses it with "great force."

THESE ARE NOT really kisses, more an erotic prelude to kissing.

Increasing sensuality
*You can make this kiss
more sensual by kissing
your partner's upper and
lower lips in turn*

THE KISS OF THE UPPER LIP

*According to Vatsyayana, when a man "kisses the upper lip of a
woman, while she in return kisses his lower lip, it is called the kiss
of the upper lip."*

IN HIS DESCRIPTION of this kiss, Vatsyayana talks about
the woman returning the man's kiss—he takes the
initiative—and the name refers to his upper lip when
it could just as easily have referred to her lower lip.
Later on in his discussion of kissing, however, he
makes it clear that kisses can be initiated by
women as well as by men. This principle
should apply to all areas of lovemaking:
women should not be afraid to make the
first move.

Positions
*Like most kisses, this
one can be given from
a sitting, standing, or
lying position*

> 66 *Whatever things may be done by one of the lovers to the other, the same should be returned by the other.* 99

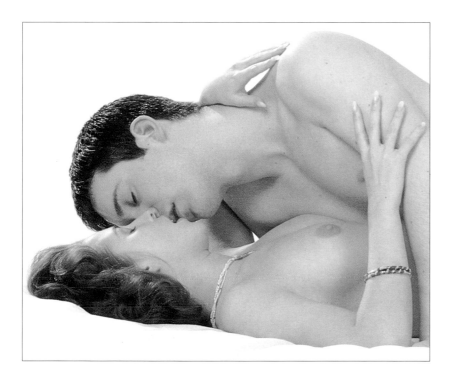

THE CLASPING KISS

◇

When either the man or woman "takes both the lips of the other between his or her own, it is called a clasping kiss. A woman, however, only takes this kind of kiss from a man who has no mustache. And on the occasion of this kiss, if one of them touches the teeth, the tongue, and the palate of the other with his or her tongue, it is called the fighting of the tongue. In the same way, the pressing of the teeth of the one against the mouth of the other is to be practiced."

HERE, WE HAVE the *Kama Sutra* describing what we would nowadays refer to as French kissing, and the author makes it clear that the initiative can come from the woman just as easily as from the man. In this type of kissing, scrupulous oral hygiene is, of course, essential.

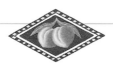

A YOUNG GIRL'S KISSES

In his chapter on kissing, Vatsyayana says that when a couple makes love for the first time, kissing should be done moderately, and not continued for a long time. He later lists the places that should be kissed, then describes three kinds of kisses that a young girl might give her partner. The places to be kissed are, he says, "the forehead, the eyes, the cheeks, the throat, the bosom, the breasts, the lips, and the interior of the mouth. Moreover the people of the Lat country kiss also on the following places, viz., the joints of the thighs, the arms, and the navel."

However, he seems to have some reservations about the kissing habits of the people of the Lat country, because he then goes on to say, "But Vatsyayana thinks that though kissing is practiced by these people in the above places on account of the intensity of their love, and the customs of their country, it is not fit to be practiced by all."

He names the young girl's kisses the Nominal Kiss, the Throbbing Kiss, and the Touching Kiss, and describes them as follows:

THE NOMINAL KISS
"When a girl only touches the mouth of her lover with her own, but does not herself do anything, it is called the nominal kiss."

THE THROBBING KISS
"When a girl, setting aside her bashfulness a little, wishes to touch the lip that is pressed into her mouth, and with that object moves her lower lip, but not the upper one, it is called the throbbing kiss. "

THE TOUCHING KISS
"When a girl touches her lover's lip with her tongue, and having shut her eyes, places her hands on those of her lover, it is called the touching kiss."

THE KISS THAT KINDLES LOVE

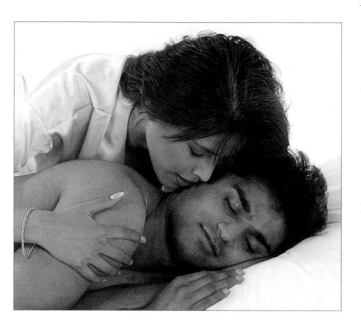

As its name suggests, this is a kiss that a woman can use to arouse her partner when he is asleep and she is feeling amorous: "When a woman looks at the face of her lover while he is asleep, and kisses it to show her intention or desire, it is called a kiss that kindles love."

FROM HIS DESCRIPTION of this kiss and of the Kiss That Turns Away, it is clear that Vatsyayana had no problem with the idea of a woman initiating sexual activity. Nearly 2,000 years later, however, many men still find it difficult to accept the woman taking the lead in lovemaking. But using seductive kisses is often a very effective way of awakening your lover and turning him on, especially in the morning. Whether or not it will work if he has fallen asleep after making love is another question.

PLAYING THE KISSING GAME

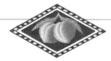

The *Kama Sutra* describes a kissing game for lovers to play: "As regards kissing, a wager may be laid as to which will get hold of the lips of the other first. If the woman loses, she should pretend to cry, should keep her lover off by shaking her hands, and turn away from him and dispute with him saying, 'Let another wager be laid.' If she loses this a second time, she should appear doubly distressed, and when her lover is off his guard or asleep, she should get hold of his lower lip, and hold it in her teeth, so that it should not slip away, and then she should laugh, make a loud noise, deride him, dance about, and say whatever she likes in a joking way, moving her eyebrows and rolling her eyes. Such are the wagers as far as kissing is concerned, but the same may be applied to pressing, scratching, biting, and striking."

THE KISS THAT AWAKENS

This version of the Kiss That Kindles Love is for a man to use on his partner: "When a lover coming home late at night kisses his beloved, who is asleep on her bed, in order to show her his desire, it is called a kiss that awakens. On such an occasion the woman may pretend to be asleep at the time of her lover's arrival, so that she may know his intention and obtain respect from him."

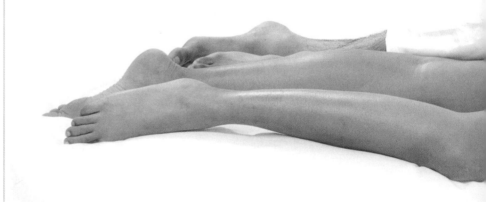

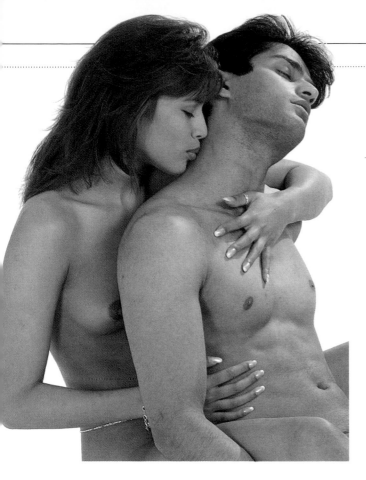

THE KISS THAT TURNS AWAY

According to the Kama Sutra, "When a woman kisses her lover while he is engaged in business, or while he is quarreling with her, or while he is looking at something else, so that his mind may be turned away, it is called a kiss that turns away."

A WARM, LINGERING kiss (or kisses) can take your lover's mind off other things and, like the Kiss That Kindles Love, direct it toward thoughts of lovemaking. If your partner is one of those men who thinks that his sexual role is to be active, and finds it difficult simply to relax and let you give him pleasure, you can overcome his resistance by following your kisses with a sensual body massage. Move on from this to a more directly sexual form of activity, such as massaging his genitals or even oral sex, and any reluctance on his part will soon evaporate.

Use your hands
Supplement your kisses with strokes and caresses

Where to kiss
Gently kiss her neck, ears, back, cheeks, and lips

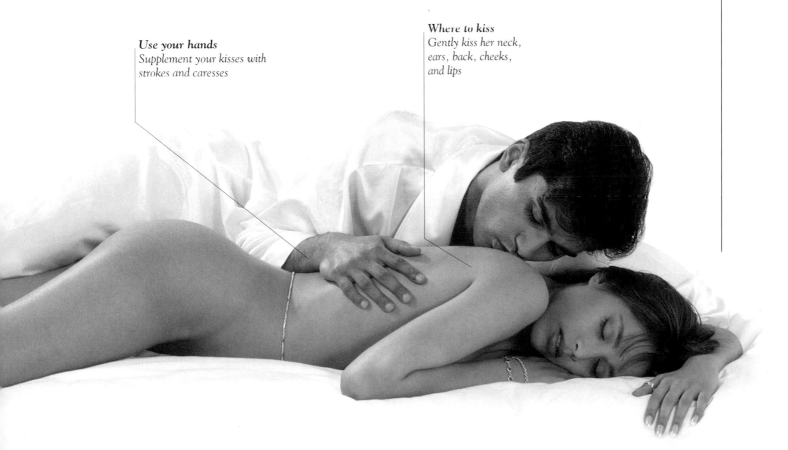

KISSING THE BODY

Although the lips and breasts are especially sensitive to the touch of the mouth, most parts of the body, including the limbs, respond to kissing; in general, the closer to the genitals, the more intense and irresistible the pleasure. There is no need for either partner to remain passive, because body kisses can be enjoyed by both partners at the same time, especially if they lie together head to foot. The *Kama Sutra*—without giving any details—says that, according to where on the body it is given, the intensity of a kiss should vary: it should be moderate, contracted, pressed, or soft.

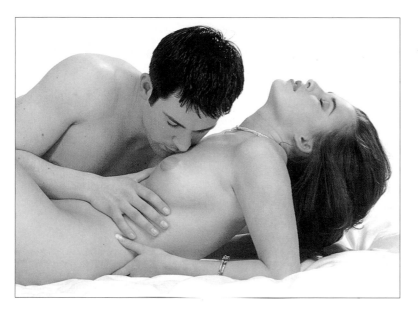

BREAST KISSING

The most effective kisses are those that are applied lightly to the fullness of the breast, while the nipples may be sucked or nibbled gently. The nipples deserve special attention, because for many women, nipple stimulation is powerfully arousing.

THE ATTENTIVE LOVER devotes considerable time to kissing and fondling his partner's breasts, because for most women this produces a response that is as emotionally satisfying as it is physically exciting. Often, if her breasts are ignored in favor of her genitals, a woman feels cheated.

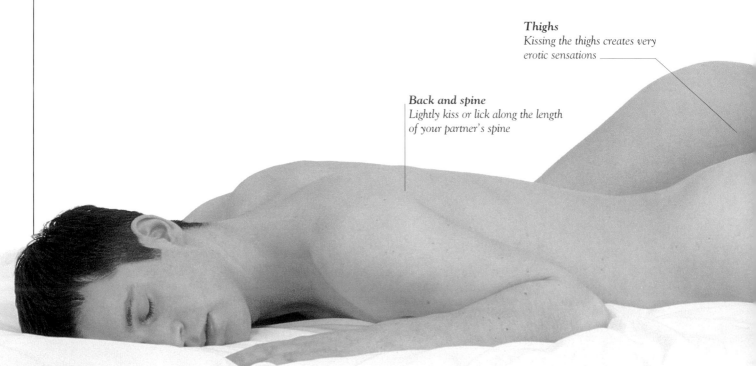

Thighs
Kissing the thighs creates very erotic sensations

Back and spine
Lightly kiss or lick along the length of your partner's spine

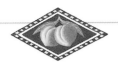

EVEN MORE TYPES OF KISSES

Among the *Kama Sutra*'s many descriptions of kisses is one called the Demonstrative Kiss. It is given when "at night at a theater, or in an assembly of caste men, a man coming up to a woman kisses a finger of her hand if she be standing, or a toe of her foot if she be sitting, or when a woman is shampooing her lover's body, places her face on his thigh (as if she was sleepy) so as to inflame his passion, and kisses his thigh or great toe."

Another kiss described is the Transferred Kiss, which is when a person "kisses a child sitting on his lap, or a picture, or an image, or figure, in the presence of the person beloved by him." A third type, the Kiss Showing the Intention, is when a person "kisses the reflection of the person he loves in a mirror, in water, or on a wall."

Kissing your lover's reflection in a mirror or elsewhere is just not possible, unless you are in love with yourself—you end up kissing your own reflection.

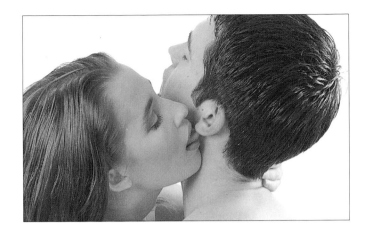

KISSING AND LICKING

Pay special attention to sensitive areas like the breasts and the nipples, the insides of the thighs, and the backs of the knees. The greater your self-control in delaying penetration, the richer the rewards when it does occur.

COVERING YOUR PARTNER'S body systematically with kisses, or exploring it all over with your tongue ("tongue bathing"), is an excellent way to heighten anticipation.

Stroking and kissing
Enhance the effect of your kisses by combining them with sensual strokes of your hands and fingers

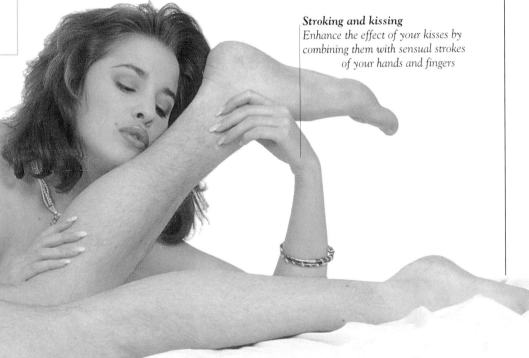

BITING

In the Indian erotic tradition, biting is an important part of the lover's repertoire, and the *Kama Sutra* catalogs the different kinds of bites in detail. Bites can be given almost anywhere on the body and range from a playful nip, more teasing than erotic, or sustained sucking that leaves a pronounced mark (today probably the most common definition of a love bite), to a forceful grip with the teeth at the height of passion. Most couples find no place in their lovemaking for this last kind of biting, and are sensible not to, because at orgasm the jaws often go into spasm and clamp shut, and can inflict a serious wound.

THE BITING OF A BOAR

For marking the shoulder, the Kama Sutra *suggests this bite, which it describes as consisting of "many broad rows of marks near to one another, and with red intervals…This is impressed on the breasts and the shoulders; and these two last modes of biting are peculiar to persons of intense passion."*

RESEARCH HAS REVEALED that women are given to biting during lovemaking, while many men feel somewhat ambivalent about it and even more so about being bitten. It has been suggested, by way of explanation, that because men are generally more muscular than women, it comes more naturally to them to express their passion through forceful bodily gestures rather than by biting.

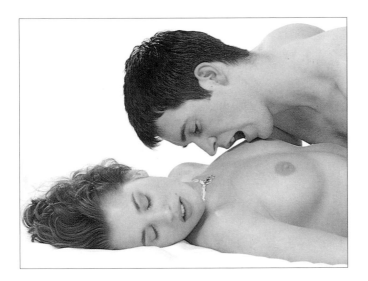

THE BITES OF LOVE

The *Kama Sutra* lists eight different types of ritualized biting for use in lovemaking. In addition to the Broken Cloud and the Biting of a Boar, these are:

THE HIDDEN BITE
"The biting that is shown only by the excessive redness of the skin that is bitten, is called the hidden bite."

THE SWOLLEN BITE
"When the skin is pressed down on both sides, it is called the swollen bite."

THE POINT
"When a small portion of the skin is bitten with two teeth only, it is called the point."

THE LINE OF POINTS
"When such small portions of the skin are bitten with all the teeth, it is called the line of points."

THE CORAL AND THE JEWEL
"The biting that is done by bringing together the teeth and the lips is called the coral and the jewel. The lip is the coral, and the teeth the jewel."

THE LINE OF JEWELS
"When biting is done by all the teeth, it is called the line of jewels."

Vatsyayana also specifies where on the face and body these various bites are to be used: "The lower lip is the place on which the hidden bite, the swollen bite, and the point are made; again the swollen bite, and the coral and the jewel bite are done on the [left] cheek...Both the line of points and the line of jewels are to be impressed on the throat, the arm pit, and the joints of the thighs; but the line of points alone is to be impressed on the forehead and the thighs."

THE BROKEN CLOUD

◇

The Kama Sutra describes this as the "biting which consists of unequal risings in a circle, and which comes from the space between the teeth," and specifies that these marks are to be impressed upon the breasts.

MOST COUPLES WHO ENJOY giving love bites draw the line at breaking the skin, preferring to suck their partner's flesh, often with the intention of leaving a mark as a token of possession. This type of ritual biting, intended to raise the skin into the spaces between the teeth, rather than to pierce the skin, serves a similar purpose.

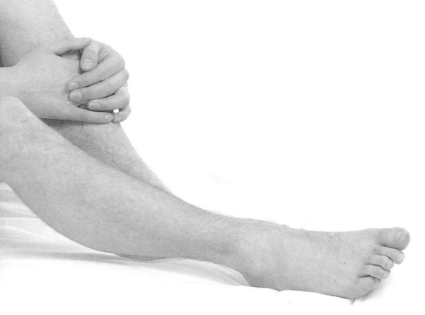

CUNNILINGUS

It is perhaps not surprising that the author of the *Kama Sutra* expresses an ambivalent, even coy, attitude to oral-genital contact. For even now, although oral sex is widely enjoyed and more freely discussed than ever before, there are people of all ages (including some who are otherwise sexually active) who disapprove of cunnilingus and fellatio, or who at least never practice them. In addition, while there are those who condemn both, there are many others who disapprove of cunnilingus but are so not so dismissive of fellatio. Their view echoes that of Vatsyayana, who concentrates on the pleasure the man derives from fellatio and covers cunnilingus very summarily. We cannot be sure what his reservations about cunnilingus were, but it is likely that the priority historically placed on the man's pleasure and the question of hygiene both played a part. Nevertheless, many people nowadays have no such inhibitions and enjoy the sensations and special feeling of intimacy provided by oral sex.

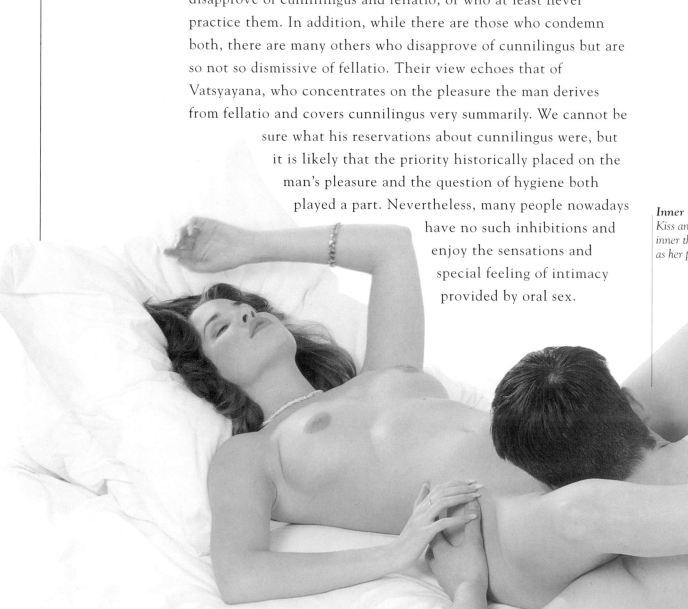

Inner thighs
Kiss and lick her inner thighs as well as her perineum

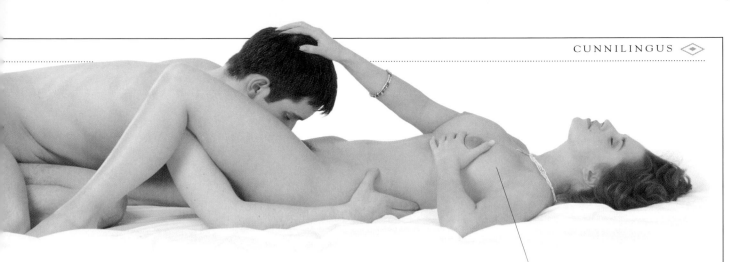

CLITORAL STIMULATION

◆

The clitoris is probably the most sensitive part of a woman's body, and it responds best to gentle stimulation from the lips and tongue. Position yourself so that you can stroke your tongue upward over the shaft and head of her clitoris. Your partner can be standing, sitting, or lying on her back; if she is one of the many women who enjoy protracted cunnilingus and can experience a series of orgasms from it, she will usually be more comfortable lying down. Stimulate each side of the clitoris in turn, always from underneath. Use featherlight strokes on the head of the clitoris, and try flicking the underside of the shaft from side to side with the tip of your tongue.

STIMULATING THE PERINEUM

◆

When she opens her legs wide, you can get between them to lick her perineum. The perineum is the area between the vagina and the anus, and in most women it is rich in nerve endings and so is very sensitive to being touched, stroked, or licked. Stimulation of the perineum can be highly arousing.

Self-stimulation
Caress your breasts and nipples to give yourself extra stimulation

CLITORIS AND PERINEUM

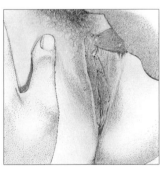

LICKING THE CLITORIS
Lick upward, and always be gentle because the clitoris is very sensitive.

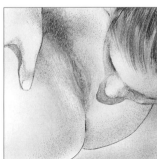

LICKING THE PERINEUM
Using the tip of your tongue, make featherlight strokes up and down her perineum.

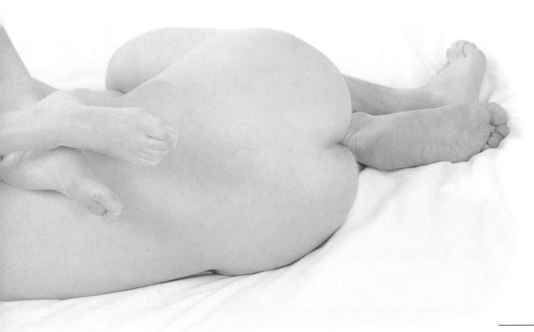

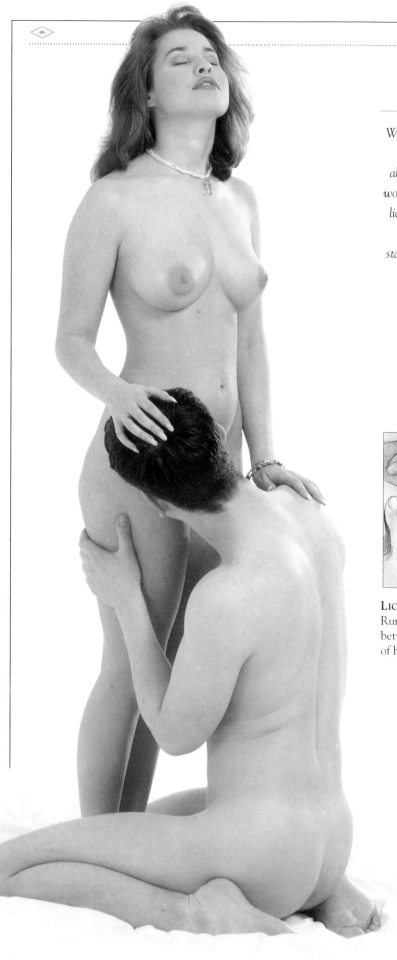

GENITAL KISSING

When you give your lover oral sex, a good way to create a slow but highly erotic crescendo of arousal is to kiss and lick her abdomen, her lower belly, and the insides of her thighs, slowly working in toward her genitals. Move on from this to kissing and licking her pubic mound, the outer lips of her vagina, and then her clitoris. A gradual approach such as this, perhaps even starting at her breasts and nipples and then working downward, helps build sexual tension, and is also useful if she is a little unsure about indulging in oral sex and needs a gentle introduction to genital kissing.

LABIA AND VAGINA

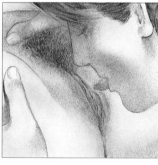 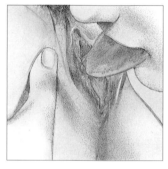

LICKING THE LABIA
Run your tongue along and between the labia (large lips) of her vagina, and kiss them.

PENETRATING STROKES
Use both deep and shallow strokes, moving your tongue up and down as well as in and out.

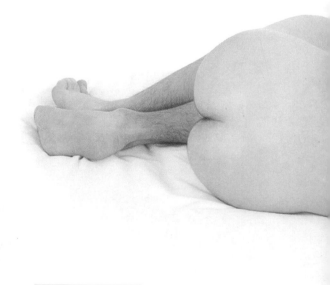

STIMULATION AND VAGINAL LUBRICATION

A woman's vagina produces a natural lubricating fluid when she is sexually stimulated, and cunnilingus is one of the best ways of stimulating her. This lubrication, besides allowing the vagina to receive a fully erect penis without discomfort, actually changes the way in which genital touch is experienced, making it pleasurable and full of sensuality. The actual stimulation doesn't have to be focused exclusively on the vagina itself, although it is usually more effective when it is. The sexiest and most erotic method of getting a woman to lubricate is through foreplay and by just turning her on.

Those women who do not produce very much natural lubricant should use one of the many water-soluble creams and jellies that are specially formulated for use as vaginal lubricants. These are inexpensive, and available from any pharmacy.

TONGUE INSERTION

After arousing your lover by kissing and licking her clitoris and perineum (see page 57), increase the stimulation by also darting your tongue in and out of her vagina. Start off by using just the tip of your tongue, then use the blade, and later alternate between shallow strokes with the tip and deep strokes with the blade. One of the secrets of giving good cunnilingus is to vary the strokes to give her an ever-changing range of sensations. Don't continue for too long with the same stroke unless she asks you to.

Relax
Lie back, relax, and enjoy the pleasure he is giving you

Hand action
Use your hands to give her extra stimulation

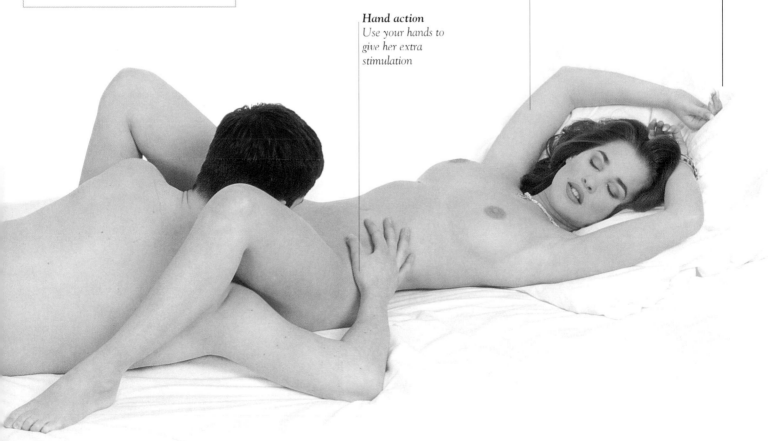

FELLATIO

While the *Kama Sutra* devotes far more attention to fellatio than it does to cunnilingus, its coverage of the former is nevertheless strange from a modern point of view. Vatsyayana describes *Auparishtaka*, or "mouth congress," as an activity predominantly practiced by eunuchs on their masters. He tells how eunuchs

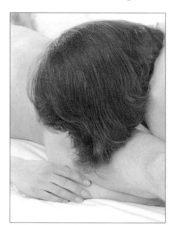

"disguised as females" led the life of courtesans, whose duties included fellatio, while "eunuchs disguised as males keep their desires secret, and when they wish to do anything they lead the life of shampooers." Vatsyayana goes on to explain how, under the pretense of shampooing (washing and massaging the body), the eunuch fondles and excites his master, eventually pleasuring him with eight kinds of fellatio, one after the other. Master and servant play a tantalizing game in which "at the end of each of these, the eunuch expresses his wish to stop, but when one of them is finished, the man desires him to do another, and after that is done, then the one that follows it, and so on."

Nowadays, gay men continue to share the pleasures of fellatio, but at the same time it is a highly satisfying complement to cunnilingus in a heterosexual relationship.

LICKING THE PENIS

Start your fellatio by licking his penis as though it were an ice cream cone. Hold its base in one hand and then, using the blade of your tongue, repeatedly lick upward, first on one side and then on the other.

Put her in charge
Try to relax and let your partner decide on how she wants to pleasure you

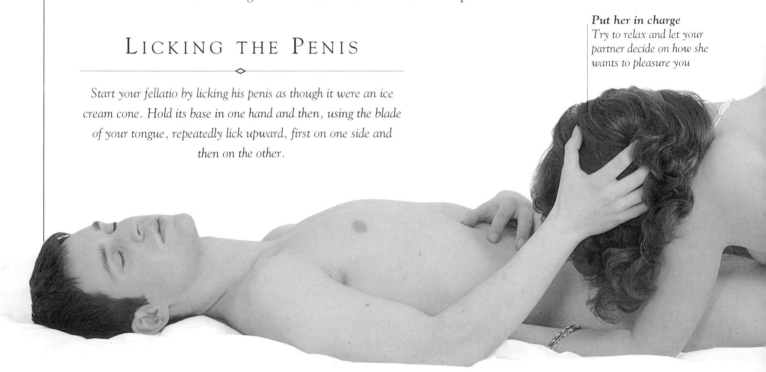

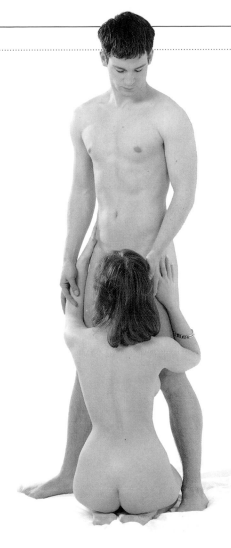

USING YOUR LIPS

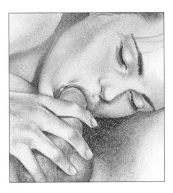

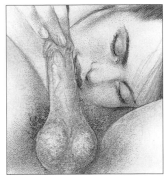

THE NOMINAL CONGRESS
Take his penis in your hand, place it between your lips, and move it around in your mouth.

BITING THE SIDES
Cover the end of his penis with your fingers, then kiss and gently nibble the sides.

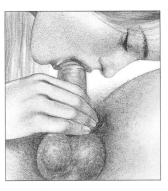

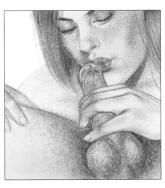

PRESSING INSIDE
Take his penis into your mouth, press it with your lips, and then take it out.

PRESSING OUTSIDE
Press your lips against the end of his penis, and kiss it as if drawing it out.

THE BUTTERFLY FLICK

This highly effective fellatio technique consists of flicking your tongue lightly along the ridge on the underside of his penis. At first, you may need to hold the base of his penis when you perform this move, but when you are adept at it, you will be able to perform it without using your hands, leaving them free to caress and fondle him.

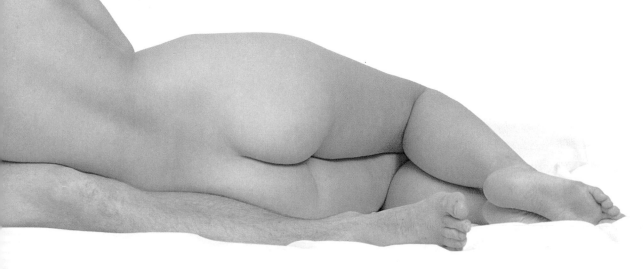

ORAL SEX ETIQUETTE

If your partner is going to give you fellatio, make sure that your penis is scrupulously clean. During fellatio, always let your partner know if you feel that you are about to climax, so that she can withdraw your penis before you do so if she does not want you to ejaculate
in her mouth.

LICKS AND KISSES

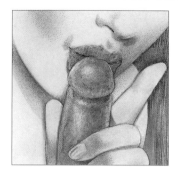 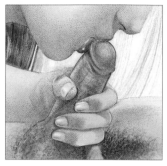

RUBBING
After kissing his penis, lick it all over and pass your tongue over its end.

KISSING
Holding his penis in your hand, kiss it as though you were kissing his lower lip.

SUCKING THE PENIS

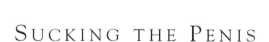

Some women want to share this intimate pleasure with their partner, but are nervous about gagging during fellatio, particularly when he becomes excited and wants to thrust. You can overcome this fear by encircling the penis with one or both or both hands before kissing, licking, or sucking the end. In this way you will be in control of the depth to which it goes into your mouth. There is no need to take in the whole penis to give your partner intense pleasure, because the glans (the bulbous end) is the most sensitive part.

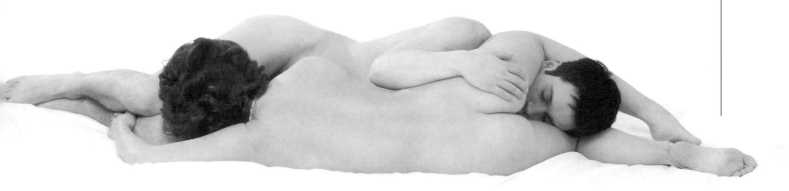

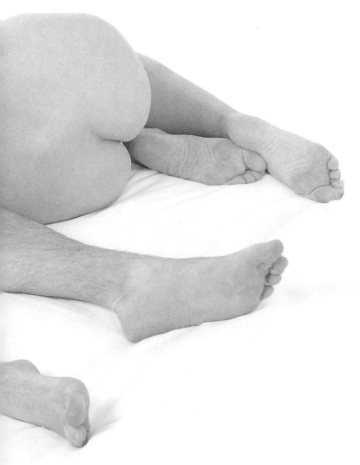

> *There are some men, some places, and some times, with respect to which these practices can be made use of.*

THE CONGRESS OF A CROW

According to the Kama Sutra, "when a man and woman lie down in an inverted order, i.e., with the head of one toward the feet of the other, and carry on this congress, it is called the congress of a crow."

THIS TERSE ACCOUNT of simultaneous oral sex in fact describes the classic "Sixty-Nine," in which the two partners perform simultaneous fellatio and cunnilingus. Whatever oral-genital stimulation lovers give each other individually, Sixty-Nine should allow them to do together. This may seem like an ideal arrangement that ensures truly mutual joy, but in reality it may prove awkward, and less satisfactory than practicing fellatio and cunnilingus in turn.

MOUTH WORK

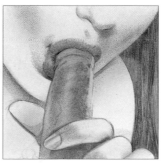

SUCKING A MANGO FRUIT
Take his penis about halfway into your mouth, and then suck it vigorously.

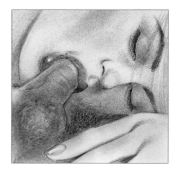

SWALLOWING UP
Take the whole length of his penis into your mouth, as if trying to swallow it.

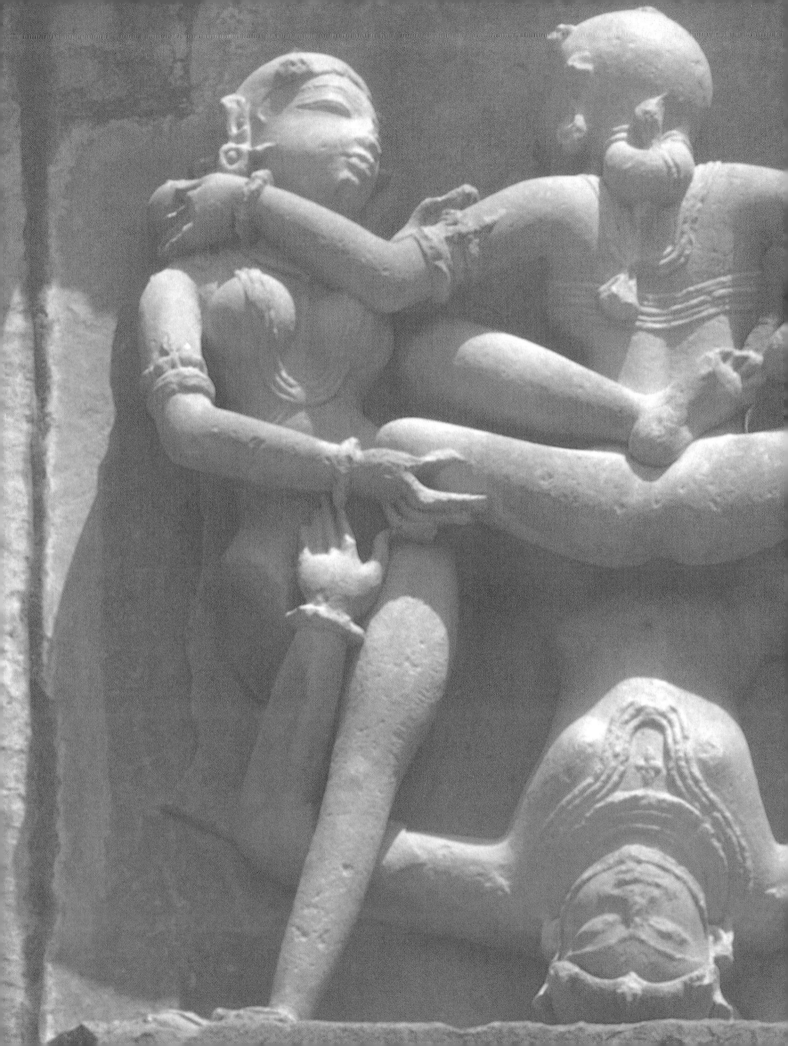

LOVEMAKING POSITIONS

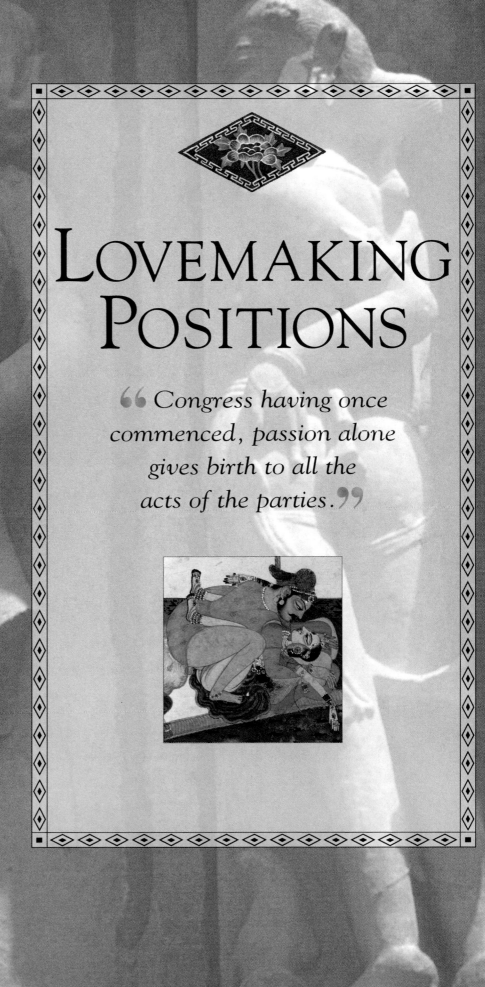

" Congress having once commenced, passion alone gives birth to all the acts of the parties. "

KAMA SUTRA POSITIONS

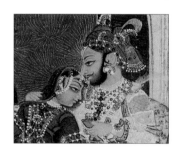

In most people's minds, the words Kama Sutra evoke a beguiling blend of the exotic and the erotic, conjuring up visions of large numbers of impractical, bizarre, or even impossible lovemaking positions. In fact, the work describes only about two dozen positions, and most of these are relatively easy to accomplish if the woman is reasonably supple. Its author, Vatsyayana, lists eight basic positions that had been described by an earlier writer, Babhravya, and attributes the descriptions of most of the rest to another early author, Suvarnanabha. Most of these sexual positions involve the woman lying on her back with her legs in a variety of postures, but later in the Kama Sutra, Vatsyayana suggests three woman-on-top forms of lovemaking that should be used when a woman "acts the part of a man." He recommends that when a woman "sees that her lover is fatigued by constant congress, without having his desire satisfied, she should, with his permission, lay him down upon his back, and give him assistance by acting his part. She may also do this to satisfy the curiosity of her lover, or her own desire of novelty."

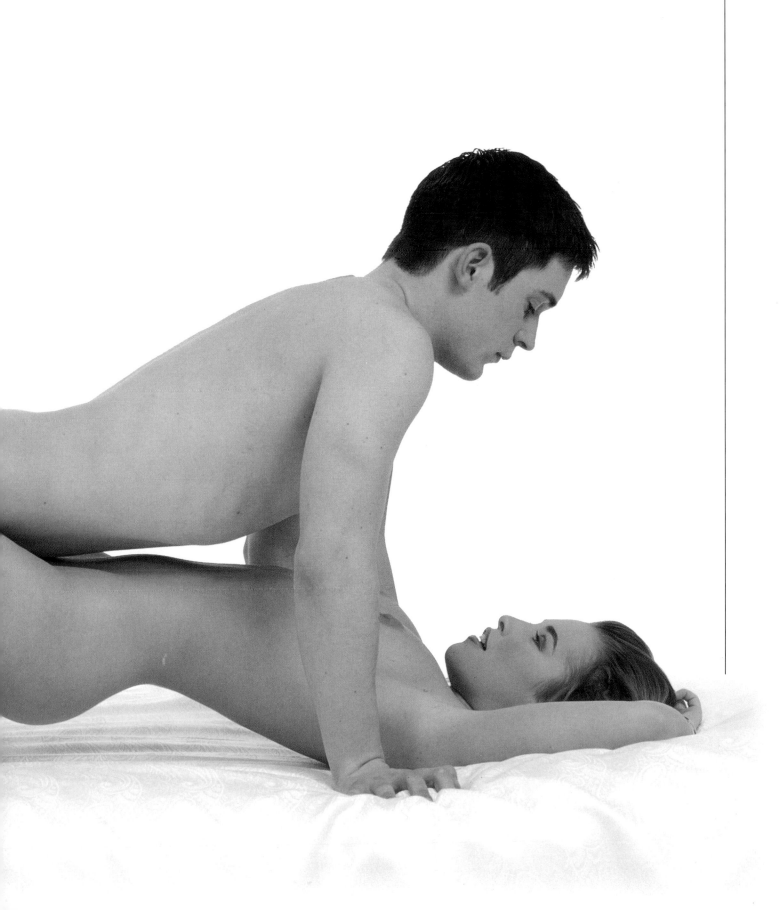

THE YAWNING POSITION

Lovemaking that begins with a straightforward man-on-top position, in which both partners' legs are outstretched, often develops quite naturally into the Yawning Position, in which the woman raises her thighs and parts them widely.

THE BARRIER PRESENTED by the woman's thighs in this position does not allow for very deep penetration, and it is unlikely that her clitoris will receive much stimulation. Offsetting this, though, is the undeniable eroticism of the position. Her genitals are displayed, and the helplessness she feels when in this position can be a powerful turn-on.

Press inward
Pressing your legs against his sides will make it easier to keep them raised

Lean forward
Gently lean forward as you thrust against your lover's thighs

Thigh angle
Changing the angle of your thighs in relation to your body is an easy way to vary the depth of penetration

THE VARIANT YAWNING POSITION

◆

The deepest possible penetration, giving intense pleasure to both partners, is achieved with this variation on the Yawning Position. Because of the extreme depth of penetration, the woman should be fully aroused, with her vagina completely dilated, before her partner enters her.

THIS IS THE POSITION you are most likely to slip into, with some relief, after playing with the Yawning Position. It is far more satisfactory, because it combines the ease of the missionary position with greater penetration and an erotic element derived from the woman's legs still being high in the air.

Foot positions
Place one foot on either side of his head

Brace yourself
Rest your calves on his shoulders and brace yourself against his body as he thrusts

THE WIDELY OPENED POSITION

◆

With her head thrown back, the woman arches her back and raises her body to meet her partner, opening her legs wide and giving an angle of entry that ensures deep penetration.

THE GENITAL CONTACT OFFERED by this position is likely to bring more satisfaction to the woman than to the man. This is because it gives her clitoris full exposure to the friction of intercourse, but he may miss the feeling of tight containment he gets when she closes her legs against his penis.

Support
Prop yourself up on your arms

Eye contact
Look into your lover's eyes to increase your feelings of intimacy

A MAN'S DUTY TO HIS PARTNER

The *Kama Sutra* places the obligation on the man to satisfy his partner, and to help him achieve this aim offers the following suggestions on movements during lovemaking:

◆ *Moving Forward*—straightforward penetration

◆ *Churning*—holding and moving the penis in the vagina

◆ *Piercing*—penetrating the vagina from above and pushing against the clitoris

◆ *Pressing*—pushing the penis forcefully against the vagina

◆ *Giving a Blow*—removing the penis and striking the vagina with it

◆ *Blow of the Bull*—rubbing one side of the vagina with the penis

◆ *Blow of the Boar*—rubbing both sides of the vagina with the penis

◆ *Sporting of the Sparrow*—moving the penis rapidly and lightly in and out of the vagina.

The man's duty as described here is very penis-oriented by present-day standards. There are, however, some good ideas for stimulating the female genitals – we have almost forgotten that using the penis as a kind of vibrator can be immensely arousing.

Thighs and buttocks
Stroke and fondle her thighs and buttocks

Bend your knees
Bring your legs back as far as you can, then bend them at the knee so that your calves press against the backs of your thighs

THE POSITION OF THE WIFE OF INDRA

◇

Achievable only by the loosest of limb, this position is recommended by the Kama Sutra as suitable for the "highest congress" —lovemaking in which the vagina is fully open, ensuring maximum penetration. Most couples who try it, however, will probably use it simply as a brief interlude between less demanding postures. The position is named after Indrani, the beautiful and seductive wife of the Hindu deity Indra. He was the king of the gods in the early Vedic writings, and also the god of rain and thunder.

I THINK WE HAVE TO assume that the Wife of Indra achieved a sense of deep sexual tension from being bundled up into a package. A woman can achieve considerable arousal by tensing her vaginal muscles, which happens when the legs are drawn up as close as possible to the body. In the buildup of sexual excitement, tension is vital. Orgasm is the relief of sexual tension, and without enough tension, it is very hard and sometimes impossible to achieve. The areas around the pelvis, in particular in the thighs and buttocks, fill with sexual tension, and it is possible to aid and enhance climax by deliberately building such tension. Bioenergetic exercises, such as flexing the thighs and buttocks or practicing the Kegel exercises (*see page 77*), can help in building up sexual tension.

> ❝ *Such passionate actions and amorous gesticulations or movements, which arise on the spur of the moment, and during sexual intercourse, cannot be defined, and are as irregular as dreams.* ❞

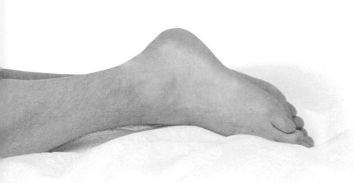

CARESSING HER BREASTS
If your partner keeps her knees parted, you can reach down to stroke and fondle her breasts. Do not attempt this, however, if it forces you to push hard against her feet and cause her discomfort.

Be gentle
Lean gently against your partner's feet, and hold on to her thighs to help you control your thrusting

THE POWER OF TOUCH

Touch is an important and enhancing aspect not only of sexual relationships but also of many other forms of human contact. For example, patients in comas respond positively to routine touch by nurses, and research shows that babies who are touched often are soothed more easily, and are likely to show better emotional and physical development, than those deprived of frequent touch.

SIDE-BY-SIDE CLASPING POSITION

For the gentle, relaxed, side-by-side version of the Clasping Position (see opposite), *the Kama Sutra suggests that the man should always lie on his left-hand side and the woman on her right, but the choice of sides is yours.*

SUCH A CLOSE, LOVING embrace is highly reassuring, especially in the early days of a sexual relationship when lovemaking can be a cause for anxiety. Just the act of wrapping yourself lovingly around your partner and keeping it at that for a while can allay any anxieties, giving a comforting, unhurried start to being sexual together. A couple in an established relationship will also find great pleasure and reassurance in adopting this position when they make love. Its gentle intimacy will allow them to express and thus reinforce their feelings of loving tenderness toward each other.

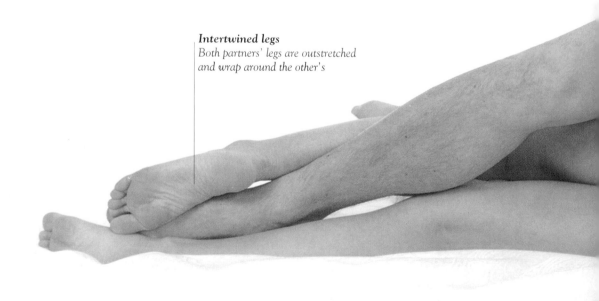

Intertwined legs
Both partners' legs are outstretched
and wrap around the other's

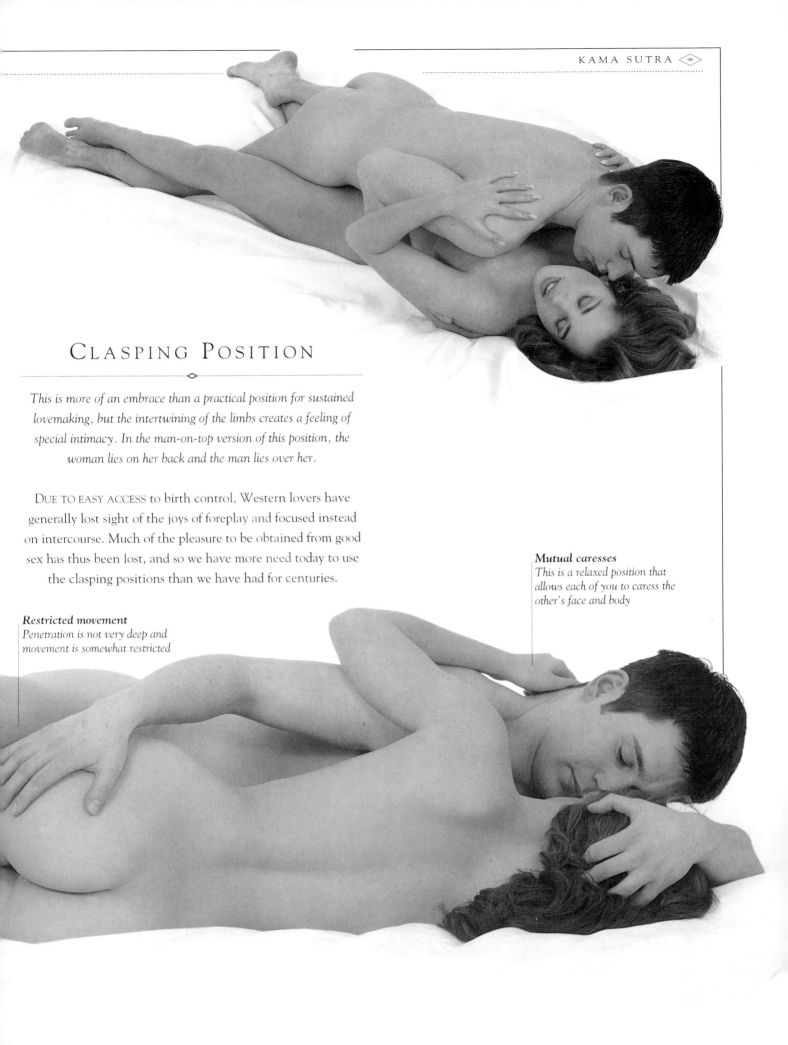

CLASPING POSITION

This is more of an embrace than a practical position for sustained lovemaking, but the intertwining of the limbs creates a feeling of special intimacy. In the man-on-top version of this position, the woman lies on her back and the man lies over her.

DUE TO EASY ACCESS to birth control, Western lovers have generally lost sight of the joys of foreplay and focused instead on intercourse. Much of the pleasure to be obtained from good sex has thus been lost, and so we have more need today to use the clasping positions than we have had for centuries.

Mutual caresses
This is a relaxed position that allows each of you to caress the other's face and body

Restricted movement
Penetration is not very deep and movement is somewhat restricted

THE PRESSING POSITION

In the most fulfilling lovemaking, as the Kama Sutra *and the other ancient manuals of love teach us, a sequence of positions unfolds in which the lovers slip effortlessly from one embrace, and one rhythm, to another, like dancers. In this way, the Clasping Position (see page 73) leads naturally to the Pressing Position. Here, the woman grips her partner's thighs with her own to tighten her vagina around his thrusting penis.*

WHAT IS WONDERFUL about spontaneous lovemaking is that it can flow like a beautiful dance where every inch of the body feels as if it is coming to life. Looked at in terms of arousal, that, of course, is exactly what happens. When the body reacts to intimate touch, the skin itself "erects" as tissues beneath it fill with fluid and muscle tension mounts. The more the partners roll around together and press their limbs against each other, the greater the sexual charge.

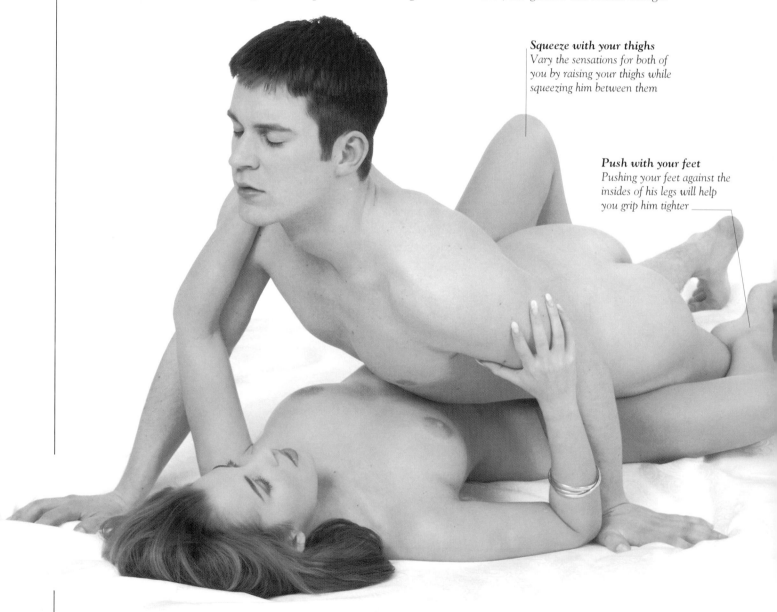

Squeeze with your thighs
Vary the sensations for both of you by raising your thighs while squeezing him between them

Push with your feet
Pushing your feet against the insides of his legs will help you grip him tighter

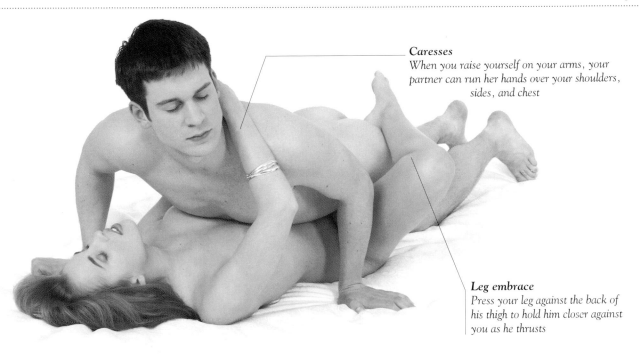

Caresses
When you raise yourself on your arms, your partner can run her hands over your shoulders, sides, and chest

Leg embrace
Press your leg against the back of his thigh to hold him closer against you as he thrusts

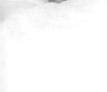

THE TWINING POSITION

Giving powerful expression to her desire to weave herself about her partner, the woman uses this variation on the Pressing Position (see opposite). She places one leg across her lover's thigh and draws him to her.

AS THE CHOREOGRAPHY of the dance progresses, the breast tissues swell, the nipples erect, the muscles begin to tense, and the labia, clitoris, and penis become erect. As both partners become increasingly excited, their chests may display a sex flush—a patchy redness under the skin, beginning from below the rib cage and spreading up and across the breasts.

THE CHAKRAS: CENTERS OF ENERGY

The idea of the *chakras* was already in existence at the time the *Kama Sutra* was written and is still very much alive today. The chakras are centers of energy that occur at seven points in the astral body, which the yogis believe surrounds the physical body. Six chakras are located along the equivalent of the spine in the physical body, while the seventh crowns the head. Sexual activity is one way of arousing the awesome energy known as *kundalini*, which lies dormant—and is therefore often depicted as a coiled serpent—at the base of the spine, in the Muladhara chakra. A person trained in yoga can direct this force from chakra to chakra, revitalizing body and spirit alike. Throughout yogic history, adherents have regarded the ability to arouse and control the flow of kundalini as a means of achieving *moksha*, or release from the cycle of life and death (the word also describes the female orgasm).

THE MARE'S POSITION

To use this technique, which can be applied in various positions, the woman employs her vaginal muscles (those that contract at orgasm) to squeeze the penis as if milking it. This produces a highly pleasurable sensation in both vagina and penis. Experimentation will reveal which positions are most fulfilling for a particular couple using this technique. For some, the best is the man-on-top Clasping Position (see page 73), but others find it more enjoyable with the woman sitting astride the man, either facing him or with her back to him.

THIS TECHNIQUE SHOWS that there is nothing new under the sun. Since about the 1970s, we in the West have been teaching young women to exercise and use their PC (pubococcygeal) muscles through the use of Kegel exercises *(see opposite)*. This helps them improve their vaginal tone after having babies, to improve their orgasmic response (stronger vaginal muscles will lead to more powerful orgasms), and to give their male partners extra stimulation.

Arousing kisses
Enhance her arousal by kissing, licking, and nibbling her shoulders and upper arms

Choice of position
When she sits facing away from you, either lean back like this or lie flat on your back

Self-stimulation
Lean back slightly to expose your clitoris for stimulation with your fingertips

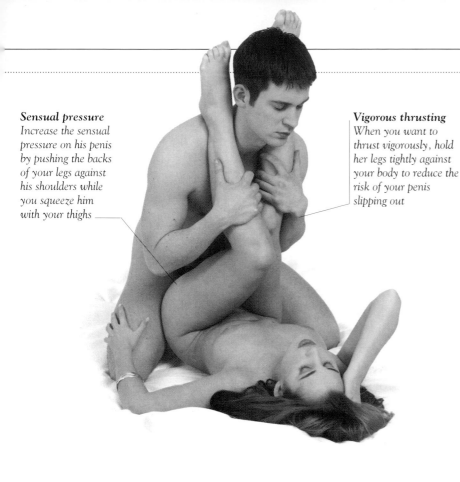

Sensual pressure
Increase the sensual pressure on his penis by pushing the backs of your legs against his shoulders while you squeeze him with your thighs

Vigorous thrusting
When you want to thrust vigorously, hold her legs tightly against your body to reduce the risk of your penis slipping out

THE RISING POSITION

◇

The woman raises her legs straight up, above the shoulders of the man, who kneels in front of her and introduces his penis into her vagina. By pressing her thighs together, she squeezes him and increases the friction as he moves inside her, producing exquisite sensations for both partners.

SINCE HIS PARTNER'S calves and feet are in easy reach of his hands, the man can either caress them or hold them to steady himself during vigorous thrusting.

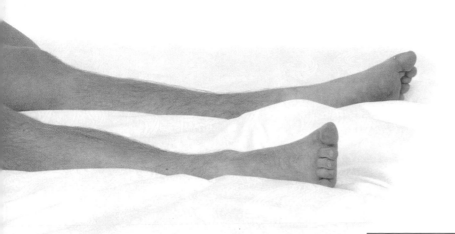

PRACTICING THE KEGEL EXERCISES

The PC (pubococcygeal) muscle exercises most commonly used to tone vaginal response are named after Dr. A. H. Kegel, the American gynecologist who popularized their use. You can do these simple but very effective exercises anywhere and at any time—in the office, in the home, in the garden.

To find your PC muscles, practice stopping the flow of your urine next time you go to the bathroom. The muscles that you use to stop the flow are the PC muscles. Practice stopping the flow several times, to get used to controlling the muscles. Then lie down, slip a finger into your vagina, and contract the PC muscles again. See if you can feel the contractions.

◆ The main Kegel exercise consists of contracting the PC muscles for three seconds, relaxing them for three seconds, then repeating. Try doing this ten times on three separate occasions every day.

◆ Do the exercise faster so that your vagina "flutters." Do this ten times, three times a day.

◆ Pretend that inside your vagina is an elevator. Your job is to move it to the top of your vagina, making three stops on the way. When it reaches the fourth and highest stop, hold it there for a while before letting it descend to the "ground floor," again pausing at each stop on the way. Try this exercise twice a day.

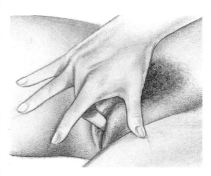

Testing your muscle contractions.

THE HALF-PRESSED POSITION

From the Rising Position (see page 77), *the woman stretches one leg straight out, past her partner's side, and bends her other leg at the knee, placing the sole of her foot on his chest. Because this position constricts the vagina, the man should take care not to thrust too hard; otherwise, the woman will feel discomfort rather than intense pleasure.*

BY STRETCHING OUT one leg, the woman gives her clitoris some chance of connection with the movement of intercourse—which she cannot do in the Pressed Position (*see opposite*) because her clitoris is tucked away between her thighs. Stretching is in itself a sexy sensation, and this may encourage the woman to move carefully under her man so that the shaft of the penis gets some extra vaginal vibration. Having one of the woman's feet flat on his chest is likely to increase the intensity of the man's feelings, just as it does when, at other times, she tenderly places her hand or head there. It can be a surprisingly loving gesture should he choose to caress her foot, possibly even raising it to kiss as a demonstration of affection.

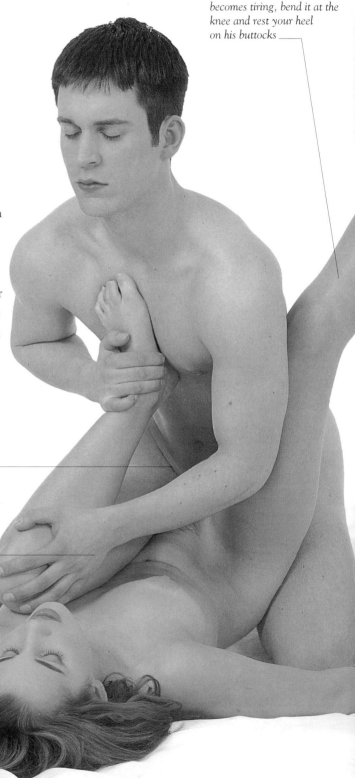

Leg angle
If holding your leg straight out becomes tiring, bend it at the knee and rest your heel on his buttocks

Vary your strokes
As you thrust, rotate your hips and vary the power and depth of your strokes

Caresses
Use one hand to fondle her foot and the other to stroke the inside of ther thigh

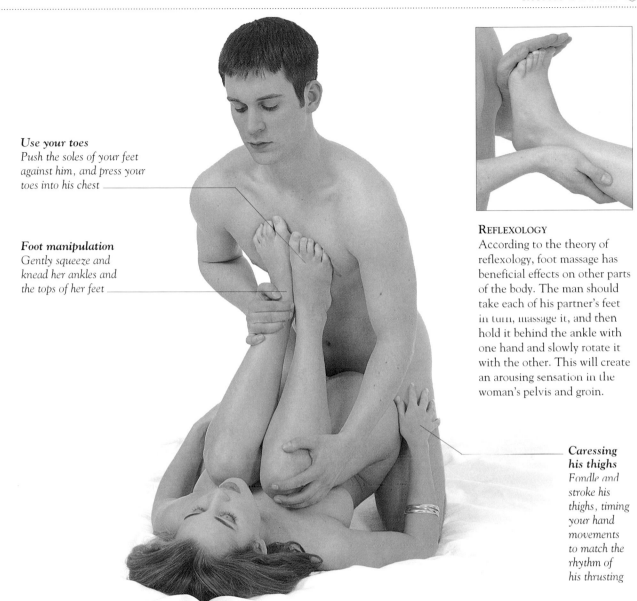

Use your toes
Push the soles of your feet against him, and press your toes into his chest

Foot manipulation
Gently squeeze and knead her ankles and the tops of her feet

REFLEXOLOGY
According to the theory of reflexology, foot massage has beneficial effects on other parts of the body. The man should take each of his partner's feet in turn, massage it, and then hold it behind the ankle with one hand and slowly rotate it with the other. This will create an arousing sensation in the woman's pelvis and groin.

Caressing his thighs
Fondle and stroke his thighs, timing your hand movements to match the rhythm of his thrusting

THE PRESSED POSITION

◇

Instead of putting only one of her feet on the man's chest, as in the Half-Pressed Position, the woman draws her thighs back to her chest, bends her legs at the knee, and places the soles of both her feet against his chest. The sensations for both partners will be subtly different from those produced by the Half-Pressed Position, but the man must find a depth and force of penetration that avoids causing pain to her shortened vagina.

THIS POSITION, LIKE the Half-Pressed, is one in which the woman assumes a submissive posture. This can create arousing subconscious emotions in both partners, enabling the woman to feel vulnerable and the man to feel powerful.

ACROBATIC POSITIONS

The lovemaking positions shown here form a sequence of rather acrobatic moves in which the woman diligently folds and unfolds her legs during the liaison. I don't think they should be taken too seriously; for example, most women wouldn't be able to assume the lotus position under normal circumstances, let alone during sexual intercourse.

THE SPLITTING OF A BAMBOO

This aptly named position calls for a simple evolution from the basic man-on-top posture, yet requires considerable suppleness in the woman. She raises one leg and puts it on her partner's shoulder for a while, then brings that leg down and raises the other. This sequence can be repeated over and over again. "Splitting the bamboo" in this way makes the vagina squeeze the penis and, whatever the rate at which the woman changes the position of her legs, it is a stimulating cycle of movements for both partners.

POSITIONS SUCH AS THIS remind me of the way young couples use their bodies and have fun inventing crazy sex positions during the early days of their physical relationship.

Lean forward
Kneel and lean forward over her, rather than stretching yourself out

FIXING OF A NAIL

◇

Instead of putting her leg on her partner's shoulder, as in the Splitting of a Bamboo, the woman places her heel on his forehead. Her leg and foot then resemble a hammer driving in a nail, represented by his head.

HAVE FUN WHILE making love—no one has decreed that sex should be a solemn business. Positions such as this are meant to be enjoyed in a lighthearted manner.

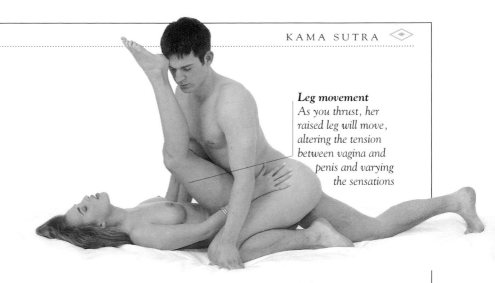

Leg movement
As you thrust, her raised leg will move, altering the tension between vagina and penis and varying the sensations

Maintaining rhythm
To help you keep your balance and maintain the rhythm while you are thrusting, hold her knees against your chest

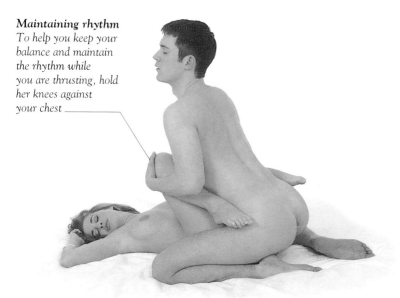

THE CRAB'S POSITION

◇

In this highly pleasurable position, which constricts the vagina around the penis, the woman bends and draws in both legs and rests her thighs on her stomach, rather like a crab retracting its claws. The man again thrusts from a kneeling position.

PLAY IS AN IMPORTANT PART of the early stages of any relationship, and play in sex is no exception. When indulging in playful behavior, for instance by adopting positions such as this, we subconsciously learn a lot about each other.

THE LOTUS-LIKE POSITION

◇

Imitating the familiar yoga position, the woman draws in her legs and folds one over the other as neatly as possible, and again the vagina is pulled up to meet the penis.

MOST WOMEN who try this challenging position find that they cannot hold it for long, if indeed they can achieve it at all.

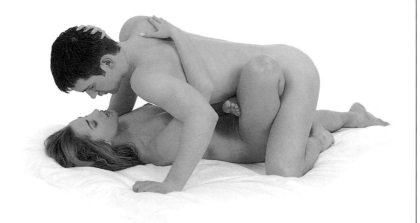

THE TURNING POSITION

When a couple is making love in the basic man-on-top position, the man can, with practice, lift one leg and turn around without withdrawing from her.

DURING LOVEMAKING, varying a position can often be used to increase the feeling of closeness. In this case, when the man turns around, his partner can demonstrate tenderness toward him by embracing or caressing his back, shoulders, and sides.

Supporting your body
Throughout this sequence of moves, you will need to support yourself on your arms and hold your upper body clear of your partner

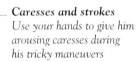

Caresses and strokes
Use your hands to give him arousing caresses during his tricky maneuvers

FIRST STAGE
The first stage in the series of moves that make up the Turning Position is to begin your lovemaking in the basic man-on-top ("missionary") position. The man should lie with both legs between those of his partner.

Buttocks
Fondle his buttocks and stroke the backs of his thighs

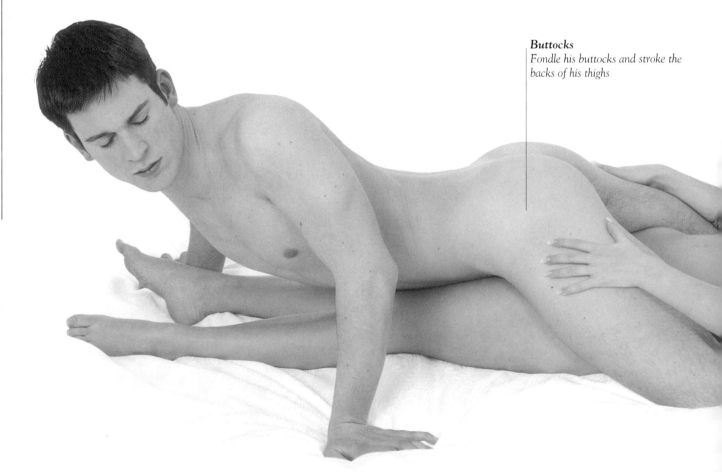

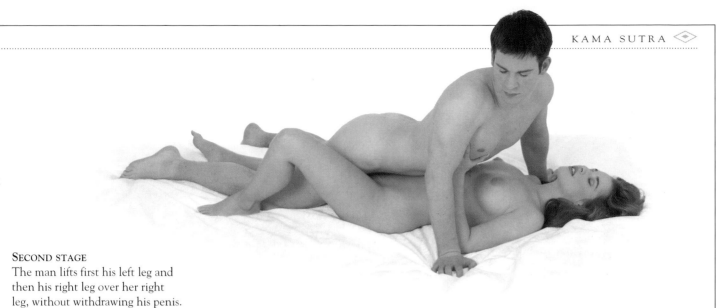

SECOND STAGE
The man lifts first his left leg and then his right leg over her right leg, without withdrawing his penis.

THIRD STAGE
He supports himself on his arms and moves both legs around, again without withdrawing his penis, until his body is at a right angle to hers.

Legs slightly parted
If your legs are slightly apart, it will be easier for him to keep his penis inside your vagina

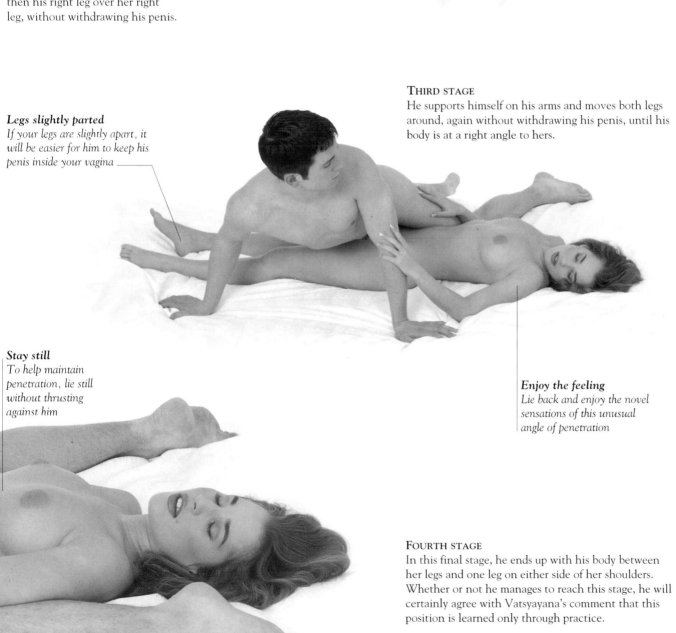

Stay still
To help maintain penetration, lie still without thrusting against him

Enjoy the feeling
Lie back and enjoy the novel sensations of this unusual angle of penetration

FOURTH STAGE
In this final stage, he ends up with his body between her legs and one leg on either side of her shoulders. Whether or not he manages to reach this stage, he will certainly agree with Vatsyayana's comment that this position is learned only through practice.

EROTIC SCULPTURES

Over many centuries, the *Kama Sutra*, the *Ananga Ranga*, and the other classic Eastern texts on love placed great emphasis on the standing positions. The special status of these positions is reflected in the fact that they appeared far more commonly than lying or sitting positions in the erotic sculptures that traditionally adorned temple walls.

Tight hold
Clasp your hands tightly together behind his neck

THE SUSPENDED CONGRESS

The man leans against a wall, the woman puts her arms around his neck, and he lifts her by holding her thighs or by locking his hands beneath her bottom.

THIS IS A POSITION THAT calls for a fair amount of strength in the man. If the woman is light, however, he may be able to support her with one arm around her waist, using the other hand to caress her.

Thigh grip
Grip his waist with your thighs and push your feet against the wall

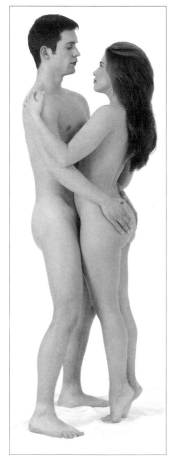

HEIGHT DIFFERENCE
Making love while standing face-to-face can be difficult if the man is much taller than the woman (or vice versa). The problem can often be alleviated by him standing with his feet apart and bending his knees slightly, or by her standing on tiptoe, but most people find it impossible to maintain these postures for very long.

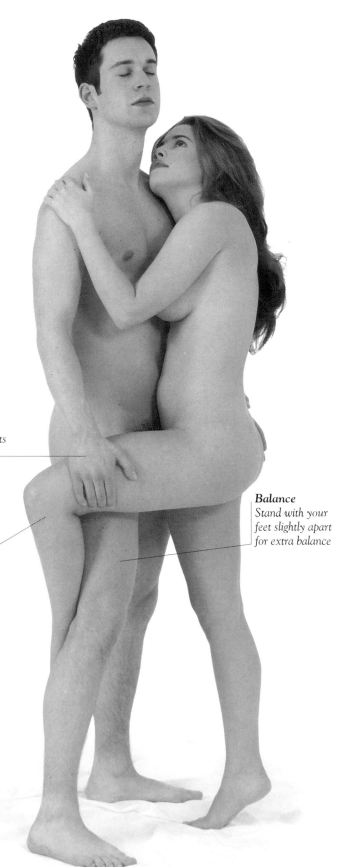

Thrusting
Hold her thigh to help control your movements when you thrust

Deeper penetration
Spread your thighs by wrapping one of your legs around his for deeper penetration

Balance
Stand with your feet slightly apart for extra balance

THE SUPPORTED CONGRESS

The lovers achieve the support referred to in this position's name either by bracing themselves against one another or by leaning against a wall.

SOMETIMES, WHEN SUDDEN passion overwhelms them, a couple may prefer to dispense with the preliminaries and make love standing up. The advantage of leaning on a wall is that with the woman firmly supported, the man finds it easier to thrust vigorously.

WOMAN-ON-TOP POSITIONS

The *Kama Sutra* recommends three movements for use when, for one reason or another, during lovemaking the woman adopts a position on top of her partner ("acting the part of a man"). She is most likely to do this either as a variation for its own sake or when her partner is tired but she is still not satisfied. Vatsyayana sees these positions as transitional, with the man eventually resuming the active role.

THE TOP

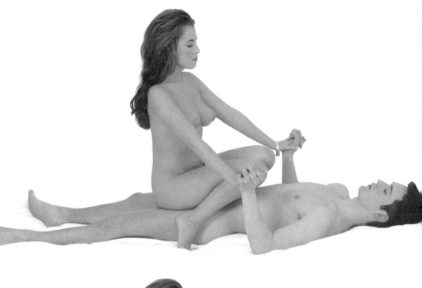

According to Vatsyayana, this movement requires considerable dexterity and is achieved only through practice. While sitting astride her partner, the woman raises her legs to clear his body and swivels around on his penis. While she is perfecting this maneuver, the woman should take care not to lose her balance; otherwise, she may hurt both herself and her partner.

THIS POSITION AND its variant, the Swing, although just about possible, really have to be the ancient Indians' idea of a joke. Most of the damage the moves could cause would be endured by the male partner. In the case of the Top, he could end up with an injured penis. This is not a position to be encouraged.

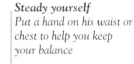

Steady yourself
Put a hand on his waist or chest to help you keep your balance

Change angles
By leaning forward or back you can change the angle of penetration and subtly vary the sensations for both of you

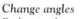

THE SWING

The Kama Sutra *suggests that, in this variation on the Top, the man should lie with his back arched. However, this is only feasible if the man has a strong back, and even then it is unlikely that he could sustain the posture for very long. It is more practical for him either to lie flat or, as here, to prop himself up on his arms.*

THE ORIGINAL version of the Swing, as described in the *Kama Sutra*, is not really a practical option, and there is a real chance of him hurting his back. The version shown here, however, is perfectly safe.

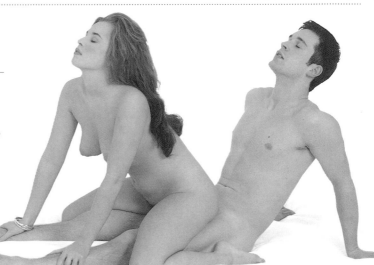

THE PAIR OF TONGS

With her legs bent at the knee, the woman sits astride and facing the man, who lies flat on his back. She draws his penis into her and, squeezing it repeatedly with the muscles of her vagina, holds it tight for a long time. Penetration is deep.

THIS POSITION IS perhaps the most practical of the three woman-on-top positions. By using her vaginal muscles (*see Kegel exercises, page 77*), the woman may stimulate her man while also arousing herself. Some women use vaginal fluttering to give pleasure, and combining this with a little movement can be a gentle method of sexual enjoyment.

> *A man should gather from the actions of the woman of what disposition she is, and in what way she likes to be enjoyed.*

THE ELEPHANT POSTURE

This is one of a number of "animal" postures listed in the Kama Sutra *and, like the Congress of a Cow (see opposite),* it is also described in the Ananga Ranga. *The woman lies with her breasts, stomach, thighs, and feet all touching the bed, and the man lies over her with the small of his back arched inward. Once he is inside her, the woman can intensify the sensations for both partners by pressing her thighs closely together.*

REAR-ENTRY POSITIONS allow deep penetration, but the *Kama Sutra* makes it quite clear that it is the association in the imagination with animals mating that gives these positions an extra eroticism. This is very different from modern thinking about animals and sex, where fantasies about a day at the zoo would definitely be considered startling.

Penetration
Pass your penis between her slightly parted legs and into her vagina

Lift clear
Support yourself on your hands or on your forearms

THE CONGRESS OF A COW

The powerful symbolism of mating animals can serve to heighten passion for many couples. In this challenging variation on the more common rear-entry postures in which the woman kneels, she supports herself on her hands and feet and her partner mounts her like a bull. It makes deep penetration possible and allows the man to control the depth and power of his thrusts.

BY EMULATING THE INTERCOURSE of animals, rear-entry positions achieve a special aspect of arousal for both men and women. Although it is much harder for a woman to enjoy orgasm in these positions, the additional stimulation provided by the man's fingers reaching around the front of her thigh to stroke her clitoris (perhaps in the same rhythm as his thrusting) can be highly erotic. So, too, can the sensation of his front pounding against her buttocks, close to her sensitive perineum and anus.

Timing
By holding her hips or waist, you can push and pull her in time with your own movements

Firm support
Keep your feet apart and the palms of your hands flat on the floor

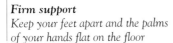

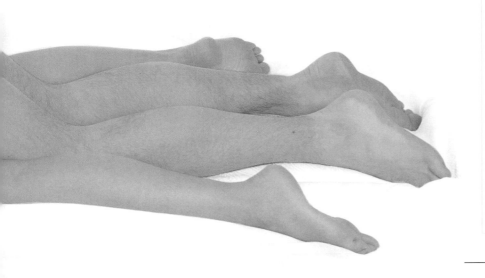

THE POWER OF THE IMAGINATION

In his chapter on sexual congress, Vatsyayana, the author of the *Kama Sutra*, implicitly acknowledges the impossibility of listing every known lovemaking position. Instead, he suggests that, by seeking inspiration from the mating habits of the animal kingdom, imaginative lovers can greatly extend their repertoires. After his description of the Congress of a Cow, Vatsyayana says that "in the same way can be carried on the congress of a dog, the congress of a goat, the congress of a deer, the forcible mounting of an ass, the congress of a cat, the jump of a tiger, the pressing of an elephant, the rubbing of a boar, and the mounting of a horse. And in all these cases the characteristics of these different animals should be manifested by acting like them."

ANANGA RANGA POSITIONS

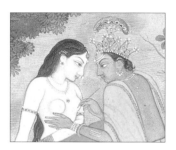

The Ananga Ranga *shares common origins with the* Kama Sutra, *but was written up to 1,500 years later, probably in the late 15th or early 16th century. Therefore, it is much closer in time to the Arabian classic* The Perfumed Garden, *although it is culturally very different. The Ananga Ranga was translated into Arabic; as a result, it exerted a strong influence on the sexual attitudes of the Islamic world. The late-medieval India of the Ananga Ranga was, like the Arab world, much more ordered than that which produced the* Kama Sutra. *Sexuality was freely expressed within and outside marriage in the time of Vatsyayana, but Kalyana Malla, the author of the Ananga Ranga, reflected a rigid society that censured extramarital sex. The major practical difference between the two Indian classics is that the* Kama Sutra *was written for lovers, married or otherwise, while the Ananga Ranga does not question the sanctity of marriage and explicitly offers instruction to the married man. Equally clear is the author's motive for writing the Ananga Ranga in the first place—to protect marriage from the sexual tedium that, then as now, can so easily set in.*

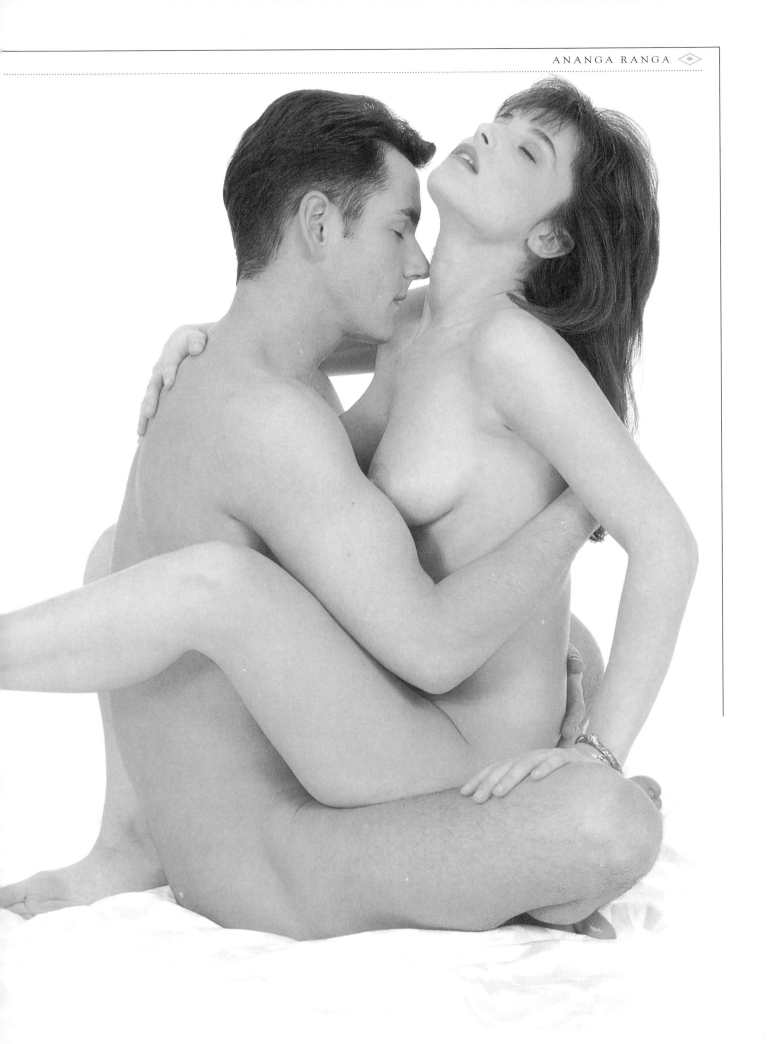

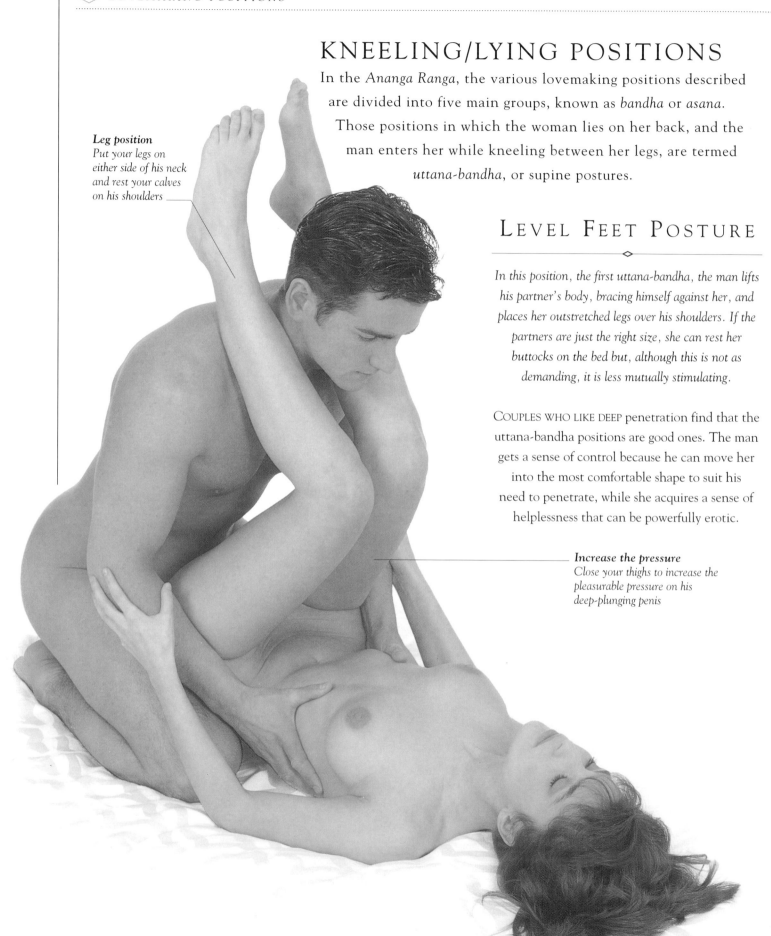

KNEELING/LYING POSITIONS

In the *Ananga Ranga*, the various lovemaking positions described are divided into five main groups, known as *bandha* or *asana*. Those positions in which the woman lies on her back, and the man enters her while kneeling between her legs, are termed *uttana-bandha*, or supine postures.

LEVEL FEET POSTURE

In this position, the first uttana-bandha, the man lifts his partner's body, bracing himself against her, and places her outstretched legs over his shoulders. If the partners are just the right size, she can rest her buttocks on the bed but, although this is not as demanding, it is less mutually stimulating.

COUPLES WHO LIKE DEEP penetration find that the uttana-bandha positions are good ones. The man gets a sense of control because he can move her into the most comfortable shape to suit his need to penetrate, while she acquires a sense of helplessness that can be powerfully erotic.

Leg position
Put your legs on either side of his neck and rest your calves on his shoulders

Increase the pressure
Close your thighs to increase the pleasurable pressure on his deep-plunging penis

RAISED FEET POSTURE

Lying on her back, the woman bends her legs at the knees and draws them back, in the words of the Ananga Ranga, "as far as her hair." Her partner enters her from the kneeling position.

BECAUSE THE MAN is kneeling, he does not need to use his hands to support himself or to maintain his balance, so he can comfortably use his hands to caress his partner and fondle her breasts. And by raising her hips with both hands, he can penetrate her at an angle that allows his penis to stimulate the front wall of her vagina, along which is located the highly sensitive G-spot.

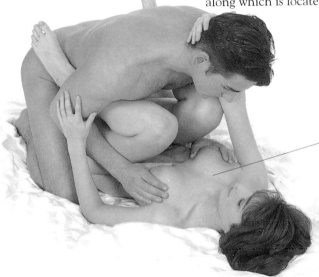

Caress her breasts
Because your hands are free, you can use them to stroke and fondle her breasts

THE G-SPOT

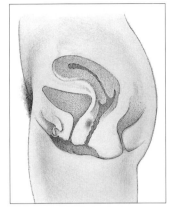

A super-sensitive area on the vagina's front wall, the G-spot is about a half to two-thirds of the way in. If pressed firmly (by the penis or a finger), it creates a powerfully erotic sensation. Research indicates that not all women possess a G-spot, but many of those who have one know that it can be capable of triggering orgasm.

THE REFINED POSTURE

Instead of resting on her partner's shoulders, as in the Level Feet Posture, the woman's legs pass on either side of his waist. This allows deep penetration, and greater stimulation is possible if the man raises the woman by using his hands to support her buttocks.

WHEN HE IS LIFTING HER and supporting her buttocks, he can apply a little gentle pressure to draw the buttocks away from the anus and perineum. This will provide her with extra erotic sensation.

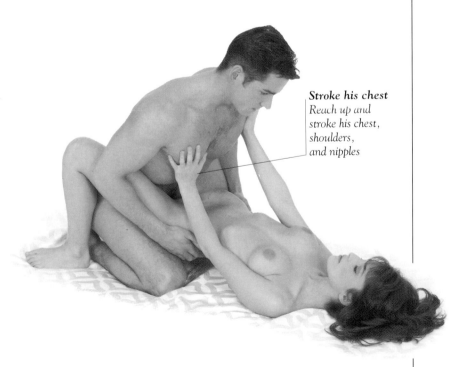

Stroke his chest
Reach up and stroke his chest, shoulders, and nipples

KAMA'S WHEEL

The man sits with his legs outstretched and parted, and his partner lowers
herself onto his penis, extending her legs over his. He then passes his arms on
either side of her body, keeping them straight. In this way he completes the
spoke-like pattern of limbs that gives the position its name.

KAMA'S WHEEL illustrates a dimension of sexuality that most of us
simply don't practice and probably find hard to comprehend. It's a
dimension that allows sex, like a type of meditation, to bring us to a
high level of awareness, a sharpness of appetite, and an increased sense
of well-being. The object of the Kama's Wheel is not to build erotic
feeling, or to achieve orgasm. It is rather to obtain a balance of mind
that feels clear, calm, and happy.

Face-to-face
This position allows
you to kiss with ease
and enjoy looking at
one another

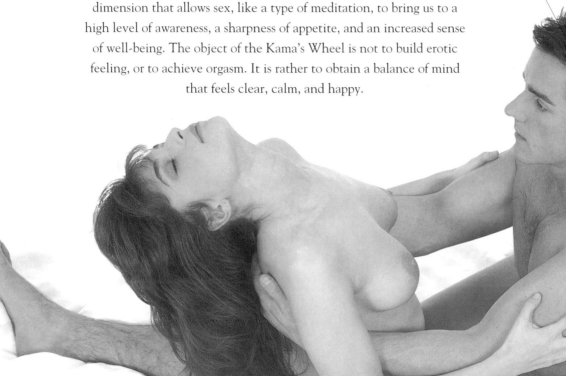

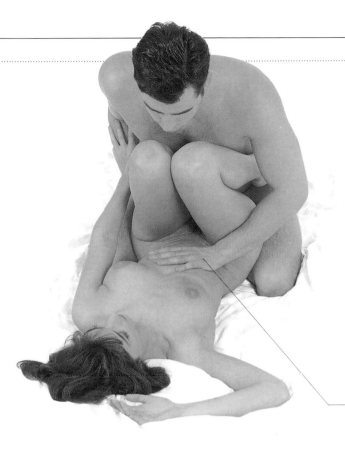

THE INTACT POSTURE

While lying on her back, the woman raises her legs and bends them at the knee, so that they rest against her partner's chest when he kneels between her thighs. Before entering her, he puts his hands below her buttocks and lifts her up slightly.

THE INTACT POSTURE IS another lovemaking position where the woman is treated like a package and the man makes the moves. If control and helplessness are important aspects of your relationship, then this could be extremely arousing mentally, although in sexual terms it is not particularly satisfactory for the woman.

Extra stimulation
After penetration, support her on your thighs so that your hands are free to give extra stimulation to her clitoris or to caress her breasts

THE PLACID EMBRACE

According to the Ananga Ranga, this position received its name from the poets of old and was "a form of congress much in vogue." The woman lies on her back and the man, kneeling, lifts her buttocks and enters her. By crossing her ankles behind his back, she can draw him closer to her and increase the feeling of intimacy.

THE OVERRIDING FEELING associated with this move is that of great tenderness. It encompasses a pure embrace in that she twines both her arms and her legs around her lover as an expression of love and trust.

Hand hold
Reach up and clasp your hands around his neck

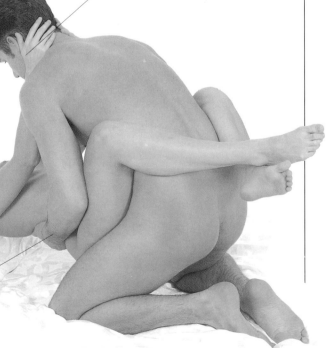

Back support
Lean forward, and slip your hands under her back

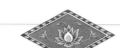

THE EFFECTS OF AGING ON MEN

It is now believed that as many as one in three cases of male sexual dysfunction is caused by physical problems, many of which are the result of the aging process. We know that the effects of aging can include damage to the arteries that supply blood to the penis, which may cause impotence. Aging can also inflict weakness of the valves of the veins that hold the blood in the erect penis, and this may cause loss of erection. In addition, it is likely that the hormonal changes that are a part of aging result in a lower sex drive and less genital sensation.

There are methods of repair and cure for some of these conditions; any man experiencing such problems should always seek medical advice.

THE GAPING POSITION

Pillows or cushions are used to arch the woman's body and to raise the man to the required height. The opening of the vagina receives strong stimulation, and for this reason some women value the position as a prelude to deeper penetration.

RAISING THE PELVIS with cushions, so that the genitals are more open than they are when she is lying flat, was a favorite sex therapy technique in the 1950s for women who didn't reach orgasm. The theory behind this technique is that if the clitoris is exposed to the thrust of intercourse, it is more likely to be stimulated. However, stimulation is usually achieved more efficiently by nimble fingerwork.

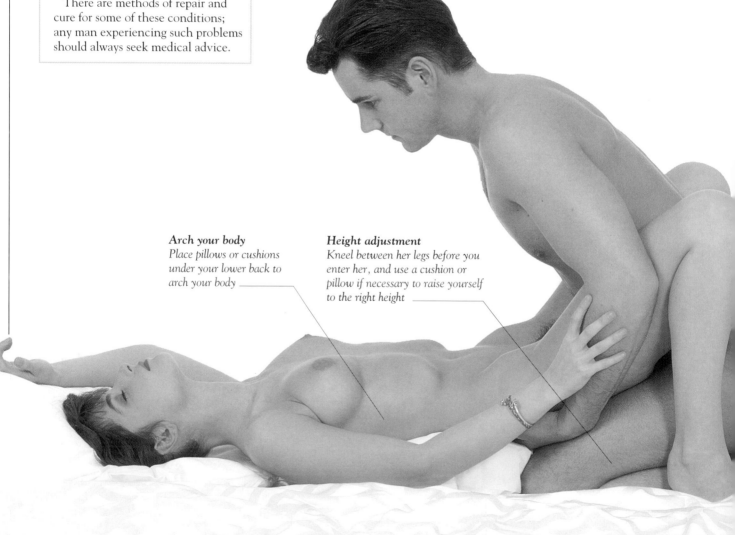

Arch your body
Place pillows or cushions under your lower back to arch your body

Height adjustment
Kneel between her legs before you enter her, and use a cushion or pillow if necessary to raise yourself to the right height

High arousal
Because your legs seem to point to and frame your vagina, the position can be highly arousing for both of you

THE ENCIRCLING POSITION

According to Kalyana Malla, the Encircling Position is "very well fitted for those burning with desire." While lying on her back, the woman raises her feet off the bed a little and crosses her calves so that her legs form a diamond shape. Then the man lies over her and enters her, as in the simple man-on-top position.

FOR HER, THERE ARE shades of bondage attached to this position, which, combined with the fact that her pelvis is opened wide and her clitoris is exposed, gives a very sensual approach to intercourse. Penetration is not particularly deep, but her very openness is an intriguing idea for her lover.

Hand support
Support yourself on your hands to avoid putting too much pressure on her crossed legs

THE SPLITTING POSITION

Increasing sensation
Keep your knees and thighs pressed close together as he thrusts, to increase the friction on his penis

Here, the woman lies on her back and her partner enters her from the kneeling position. He then lifts her legs straight up, resting them on his shoulder.

POSITIONS SUCH AS THIS are excellent for the older man who needs a more robust sensation during intercourse. His penis is snugly contained by her vagina, and the extra gripping sensation of her thighs gives the additional friction that he needs to bring him to orgasm.

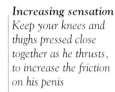

SIDE-BY-SIDE POSITIONS

The *Ananga Ranga* describes three positions in which the woman lies on her side with her partner facing her. These are termed *tiryak-bandha*, or transverse positions, and two of them are shown here; in the third, the Cupped Position, the lovers lie with their legs out straight.

THE CRAB EMBRACE

In this warm and inviting variation on the basic side-by-side position, the man enters the woman and lies between her thighs. One of her legs remains beneath his, and she passes the other over his body, just below his chest.

PENETRATION IS DEEP, but the man's movements may be restricted. Like all the side-by-side positions, it is useful when either partner is tired but still passionate. When describing a side-by-side position, the *Kama Sutra* says that the man should lie on his left side and the woman on her right. This rule is not mentioned by Kalyana Malla, but the suggestion was no doubt prompted by the fact that, then as now, most men were right-handed. However, if the man is left-handed and wants to caress his partner with that hand, or if the woman wants to caress her partner with her right hand, it makes sense to reverse the position.

Loving caresses
Use your free hands to caress each other's arms, face, torso, buttocks, and thighs

Leg position
Put your uppermost leg over his body, and rest the back of your knee on his hip

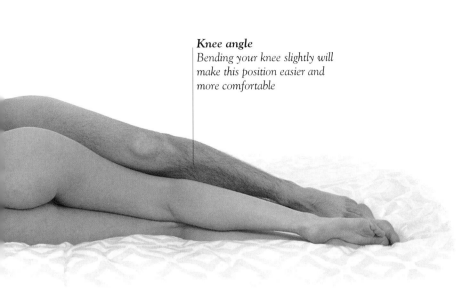

Knee angle
Bending your knee slightly will make this position easier and more comfortable

THE TRANSVERSE LUTE

◇

The lovers lie side by side with their legs outstretched. After the woman has raised one leg slightly to allow her partner to enter her, he raises one leg and rests it on her thigh.

SIDE-BY-SIDE POSITIONS are excellent for men who need more friction during intercourse. The penis thrusts are felt along the insides of the labia, which are pressed against the penis by the legs, so these positions also give the woman an increased likelihood of arousal and orgasm. And if the man pulls himself up a little higher in relation to the woman's body (that is, toward her head), he can ensure that his penis brushes against her clitoris. These positions are often used as part of sex therapy for women who have had difficulty achieving orgasms.

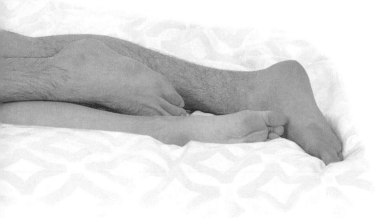

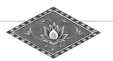

THE FOUR ORDERS OF WOMEN—PART 1

Kalyana Malla, the author of the *Ananga Ranga*, divided women into four types, according to their temperament. The first two of these Four Orders of Women are the Padmini and the Chitrini.

THE PADMINI
"She in whom the following signs and symptoms appear is called Padmini, or Lotus-woman. Her face is pleasing as the full moon; her body, well clothed with flesh, is soft as the Shiras [a tall fragrant tree] or mustard flower; her skin is fine, tender, and fair as the yellow lotus, never dark-colored, though resembling, in the effervescence and purple light of her youth, the cloud about to burst. Her Yoni [vulva] resembles the opening lotus bud, and her Love-seed (Kama-salila, the water of life) is perfumed like the lily that has newly burst. She walks with swan-like gait, and her voice is low and musical as the note of the Kokila bird [the Indian cuckoo]; she delights in white raiment, in fine jewels, and in rich dresses."

THE CHITRINI
"The Chitrini, or Art-woman, is of middle size, neither short nor tall, with bee-black hair; thin, round, shell-like neck; tender body; waist lean-girthed as the lion's; hard, full breasts; well-turned thighs and heavily made hips. The hair is thin about the Yoni, the Mons Veneris being soft, raised, and round. The Kama-salila (love-seed) is hot, and has the perfume of honey, producing from its abundance a sound during the venereal rite. Her eyes roll, and her walk is coquettish, like the swing of an elephant."

The Kama-salila mentioned in these descriptions is the woman's vaginal secretions, which were thought to be the female counterpart of the male's semen.

SITTING POSITIONS

The following six positions are forms of what the *Ananga Ranga* terms *upavishta*, or sitting posture.

THE LOTUS POSITION

In this most straightforward of sitting positions, which Kalyana Malla describes as a favorite, the man sits cross-legged and the woman sits on his lap, facing him, and lowers herself onto his penis. The Ananga Ranga suggests that the man place his hands on his partner's shoulders, but he can just as comfortably, and perhaps more affectionately, put his arms around her body or about her neck.

THE SITTING POSITIONS can be friendly, charged with eroticism, youthful, comic, acrobatic, or fun, depending on your frame of mind. They are mainly positions with which to give the male a treat, for it is the woman who tends to do all the work. One of the great strengths of the Indian love texts, however, is that although they always appear to be written from a male point of view, they are very fair, given their era, in paying attention to the sexual needs of both partners.

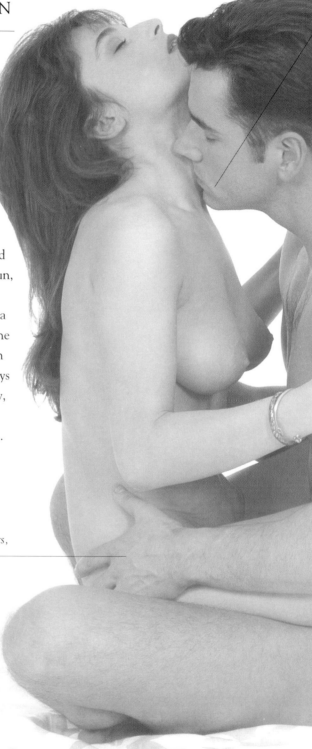

Passionate kisses
Give her arousing kisses on her throat and breasts

Caresses
Use your hands to stroke each other's neck, shoulders, arms, and back

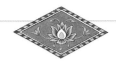

THE FOUR ORDERS OF WOMEN—PART 2

The last of the Four Orders of Women are the Shankhini and the Hastini.

THE SHANKHINI
"The Shankhini, or Conch-woman, is of bilious temperament, her skin being always hot and tawny, or dark yellow-brown; her body is large, her waist thick, and her breasts small. Her Yoni is ever moist with Kama-salila, which is distinctly salt, and the cleft is covered with thick hair."

THE HASTINI
"The Hastini [the Elephant-woman] is short of stature; she has a stout, coarse body, and her skin, if fair, is of dead white. Her hair is tawny, her lips are large; her voice is harsh, choked, and throaty, and her neck is bent. Her gait is slow, and she walks in a slouching manner; often the toes of one foot are crooked. Her Kama-salila has the savor of the juice that flows in spring from the elephant's temples."

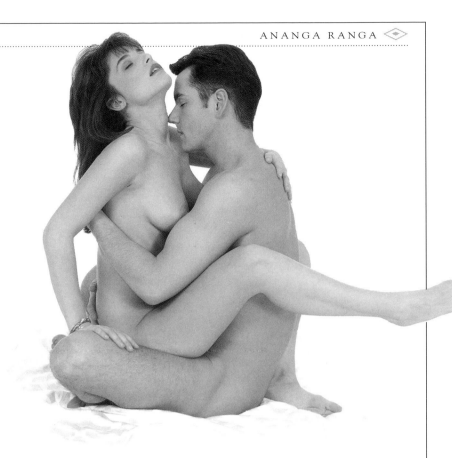

Bend your knees
Sit with your knees bent and your feet flat on the bed

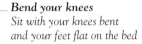

THE ACCOMPLISHING POSITION

◇

This variation on the Lotus Position requires the woman to raise one leg slightly, perhaps using her hand to help her keep her balance. Having one leg raised changes the tension between her vagina and his penis.

LIKE THE OTHER face-to-face positions, this one allows the couple to kiss and the man to fondle the woman's breasts. However, the man's thrusting movements are restricted.

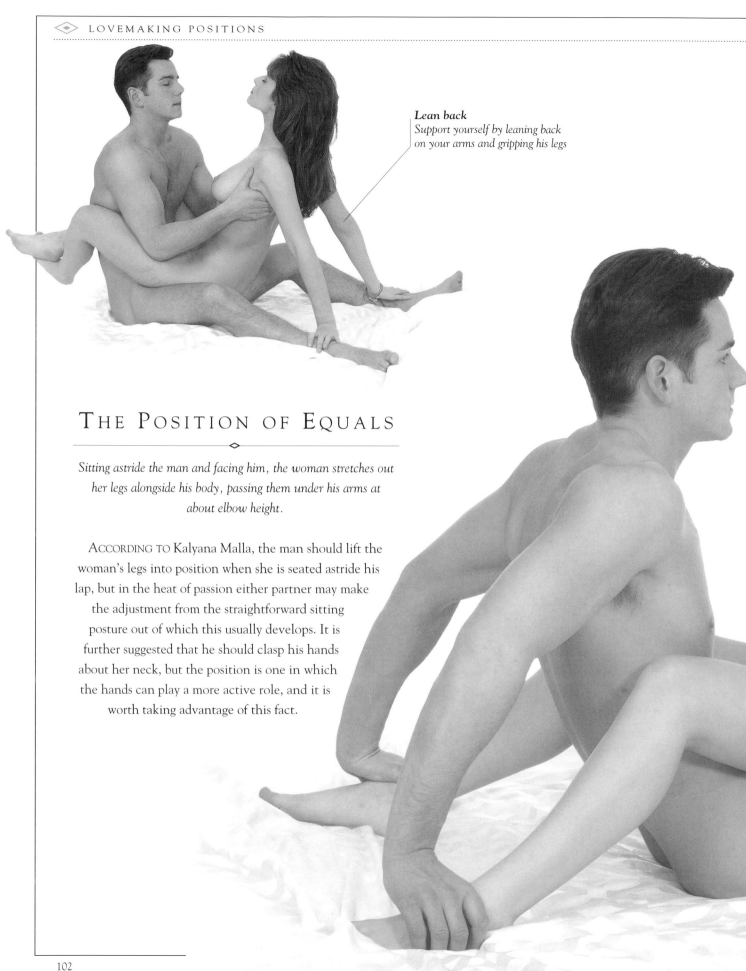

Lean back
Support yourself by leaning back on your arms and gripping his legs

THE POSITION OF EQUALS

◇

Sitting astride the man and facing him, the woman stretches out her legs alongside his body, passing them under his arms at about elbow height.

ACCORDING TO Kalyana Malla, the man should lift the woman's legs into position when she is seated astride his lap, but in the heat of passion either partner may make the adjustment from the straightforward sitting posture out of which this usually develops. It is further suggested that he should clasp his hands about her neck, but the position is one in which the hands can play a more active role, and it is worth taking advantage of this fact.

THE SNAKE TRAP

In this position, the woman sits astride the man, facing him, and each partner holds the other's feet. This arrangement allows the couple to rock themselves back and forth in a stimulating seesaw-like movement but, since it restricts thrusting, it is best adopted when the man is tired, or is satisfied and is making love again for his partner's pleasure.

BOTH OF THE POSITIONS on this page are examples of play. There is no way in which they serve any real purpose with regard to sexual stimulation, but they can be delightful for just "fooling around."

Eye contact
You can either maintain loving eye contact, or watch the action "down below"

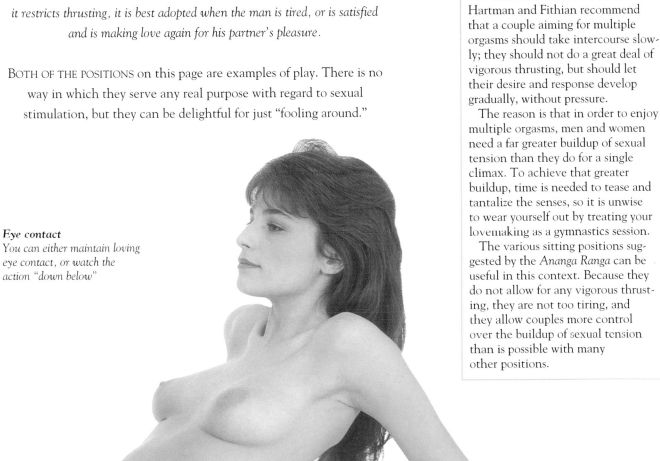

SEXUAL TENSION AND MULTIPLE ORGASMS

The American sex researchers Hartman and Fithian recommend that a couple aiming for multiple orgasms should take intercourse slowly; they should not do a great deal of vigorous thrusting, but should let their desire and response develop gradually, without pressure.

The reason is that in order to enjoy multiple orgasms, men and women need a far greater buildup of sexual tension than they do for a single climax. To achieve that greater buildup, time is needed to tease and tantalize the senses, so it is unwise to wear yourself out by treating your lovemaking as a gymnastics session.

The various sitting positions suggested by the *Ananga Ranga* can be useful in this context. Because they do not allow for any vigorous thrusting, they are not too tiring, and they allow couples more control over the buildup of sexual tension than is possible with many other positions.

THE PAIRED FEET POSITION

◇

The man sits with his legs wide apart while the woman lowers herself onto him, with her legs over his. When full penetration has been achieved, he presses her thighs together.

NEITHER PARTNER CAN move very much in this position, but the pressure of the woman's thighs constricts her vagina, producing pleasurable sensations for man and woman alike. A further benefit is the feeling of intimacy that characterizes all the face-to-face sitting positions.

Thigh stroking
Gently stroke and squeeze her thighs while you are pressing them together

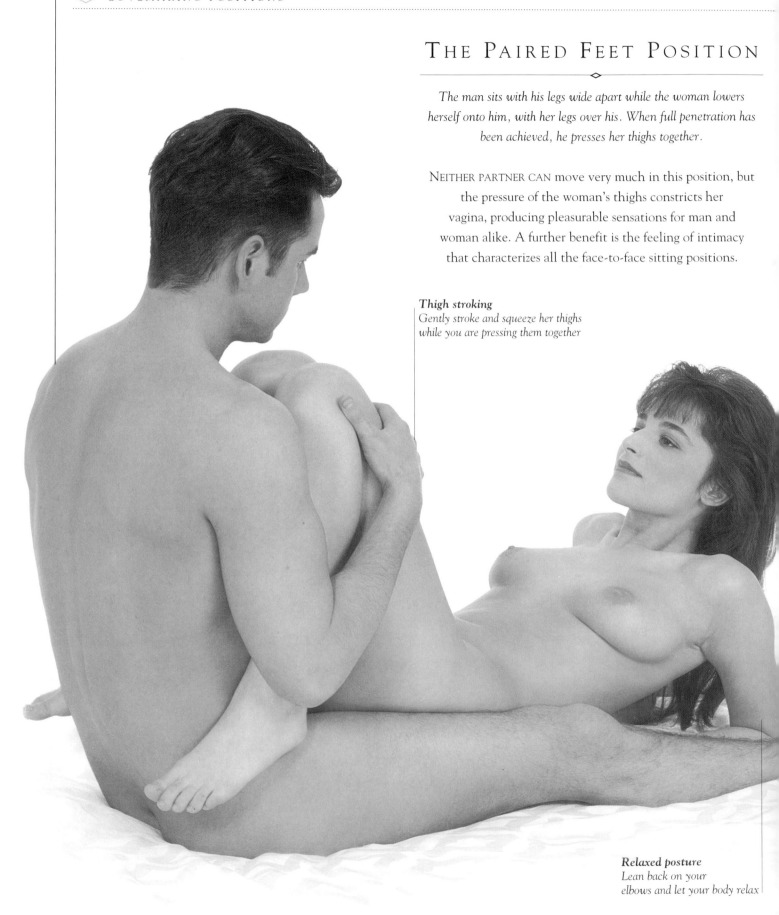

Relaxed posture
Lean back on your elbows and let your body relax

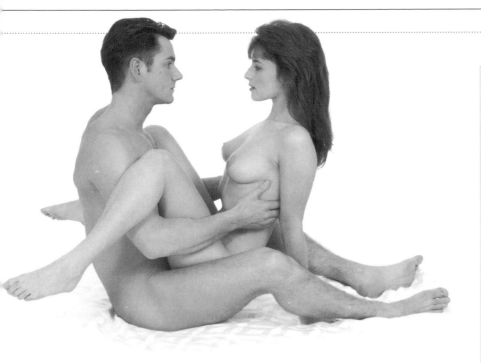

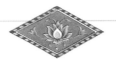

THE CRYING OUT POSITION

The man lifts the woman by passing her legs over his arms at the elbow, and moves her from side to side. In a variation known as the Monkey Position, the man moves the woman backward and forward rather than from side to side.

BECAUSE THE MAN HAS to lift the woman and move her around on his penis, this position is best, perhaps only, suited to a strong man and a light woman.

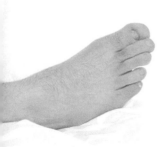

THE THREE ORDERS OF MEN

Just as Kalyana Malla divided women into four types, so he divided men into three: the Shasha, or Hare-man; the Vrishabha, or Bull-man; and the Ashwa, or Horse-man.

THE SHASHA

"The Shasha is known by a Linga [penis] that in erection does not exceed six finger-breadths, or about three inches [7.6 cm]. His figure is short and spare but well-proportioned in shape and make; he has small hands, knees, feet, loins and thighs, the latter being darker than the rest of the skin. His features are clear and well proportioned; his face is round, his teeth are short and fine, his hair is silky, and his eyes are large and well opened. He is humble in his demeanor; his appetite for food is small, and he is moderate in his carnal desires. Finally, there is nothing offensive in his Kama-salila or semen."

THE VRISHABHA

"The Vrishabha is known by a Linga of nine fingers in length or four inches and a half [11.4 cm]. His body is robust and tough, like that of a tortoise; his chest is fleshy, his belly is hard, and the frogs [insides] of the upper arms are turned so as to be brought in front. His disposition is cruel and violent, restless and irascible; his Kama-salila is ever ready."

THE ASHWA

"The Ashwa is known by a Linga of twelve fingers or about six inches [15 cm] long. He is tall and large-framed, but not fleshy, and his delight is in big and robust women, never in those of delicate form. He is reckless in spirit, passionate and covetous, gluttonous, volatile, lazy, and full of sleep. He cares little for the venereal rite, except when the spasm approaches. His Kama-salila is copious, salt, and goat-like."

WOMAN-ON-TOP POSITIONS

The *Ananga Ranga* gives details of three woman-on-top positions for use when the man is tired or when he has not satisfied his partner. These positions are termed *purushayita-bandha*, or role-reversal positions, and are fascinating because they make it clear that women's sexual needs were seen to be as important as those of men. The methods suggested demonstrate an informed awareness of how a woman's sexual response differs from that of a man. They are the forerunners of techniques that are advocated by modern sex therapists.

Comfort
*Put a pillow under your head
to make yourself more
comfortable while you watch
her making love to you*

THE ORGASMIC ROLE-REVERSAL

Kalyana Malla likens the woman's posture in this position to that of a "large bee" and asserts that she "thoroughly satisfies herself." She squats on the man's thighs, then inserts his penis, closes her legs firmly, and adopts a churning motion.

BECAUSE OF THE freedom of movement that this position gives to the woman, she can control the speed, angle, and amount by which she moves her pelvis in circles and from side to side. She can also add extra variety to the sensations she feels by varying the depth of penetration.

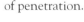

THE ASCENDING POSITION

◇

For the woman whose "passion has not been gratified by previous copulation," the Ananga Ranga recommends the Ascending Position. Sitting cross-legged on the man's thighs, she should "seize" his penis and insert it into her vagina, then move herself up and down.

AS IN SIMILAR POSITIONS, the woman can alter the angle of her partner's penis to give herself the kind of stimulation she wants; in particular, she can ensure that the G-spot (*see page 93*) receives attention. She can also stimulate her clitoris, and this, combined with her movement on the penis, may well be enough to bring her to orgasm.

Extra stimulation
While she stimulates her clitoris, enhance her arousal by caressing her thighs

THE INVERTED EMBRACE

◇

The man lies on his back. The woman lies on top of him and inserts his penis. Pressing her breast to his and steadying herself by gripping his waist, she moves her hips in every direction.

LIKE THE OTHER woman-on-top positions shown here, the Inverted Embrace puts her in control of the movements of lovemaking. The feeling of power that this gives can increase her excitement—just as the man's pleasure can be increased if he is not afraid of relinquishing control.

PERFUMED GARDEN POSITIONS

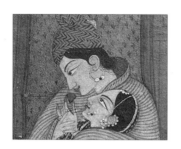

In the male-dominated, North African culture of the late 15th century in which it was written, Sheikh Nefzawi's The Perfumed Garden would have been regarded as something to be hidden away from the womenfolk, a manual of practical advice with which they had no need to concern themselves. It provided ample instruction, often in highly poetic and evocative language, on what a man could do to and with his wife or mistress, but barely touched on her experience. Even though its outlook feels dated, and perhaps even alien, The Perfumed Garden goes to the heart of the matter, explaining a wealth of positions and techniques that will, in fact, deepen the experience of lovemaking for man and woman alike. As more and more women are freeing themselves from the sexual stereotyping that has traditionally turned them into mere objects of men's desire, many are actively seeking ways in which to increase their own sexual pleasure. For them, the primary goal is to cast off the passive role and feel free to decide with their partners what they want from sex. Exploring the positions on the following pages, all inspired by The Perfumed Garden, should form part of that quest. The Perfumed Garden describes 11 main lovemaking postures, and these are followed by many more positions, including some from India and other cultures.

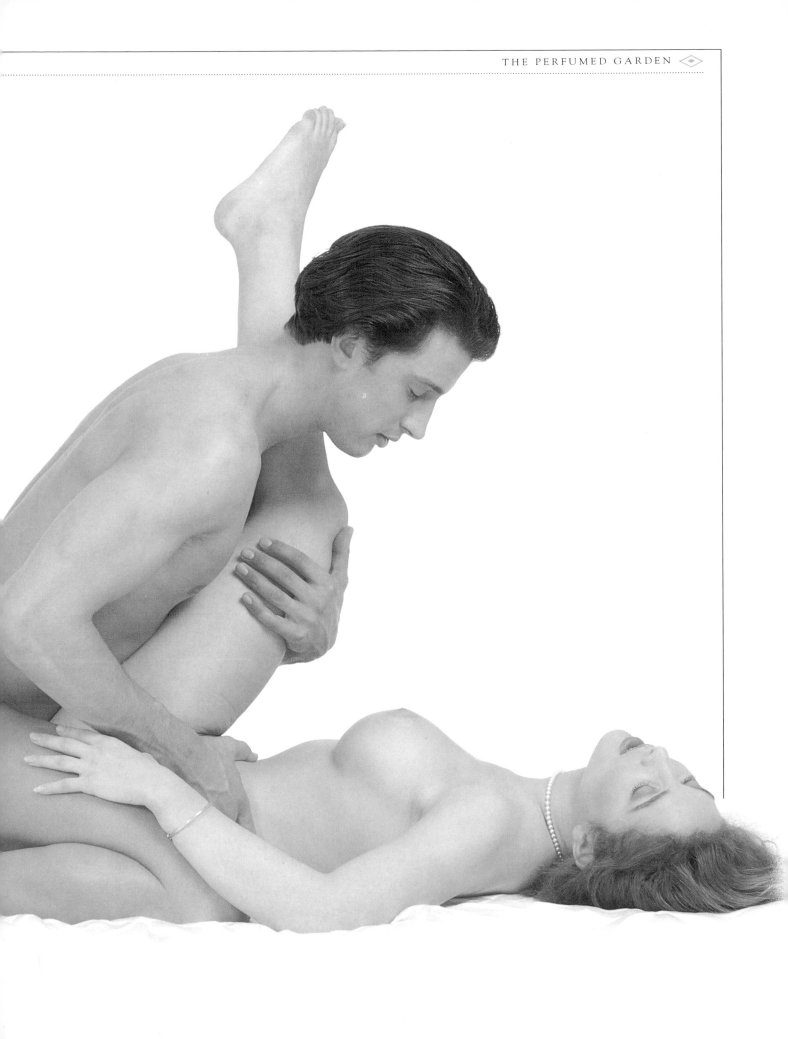

FIRST POSTURE

◆

A straightforward man-on-top position, the First Posture is said by Sheikh Nefzawi to be particularly suitable for the man with a long penis.

I THINK SHEIKH NEFZAWI is in many ways nearer to being a sex therapist than any of the other ancient authors featured in this book, and he makes sensible allowances for physical differences between men and women. Here, for example, he has selected a classic position in which a man with a long penis could easily adjust his length of thrust so as not to hurt his partner. This is a very real consideration when the man and the woman are of greatly differing builds.

Thigh position
Lie on your back and raise your thighs before he enters you

Controlled thrusting
When you have entered her, support yourself on your hands and grip the bed with your toes to help you control the rhythm and depth of your thrusting

SECOND POSTURE

◆

This can hardly be described as a comfortable position for the woman, but Sheikh Nefzawi, undeterred, recommends its use to the man whose "member is a short one."

Easier entry
By drawing your out-stretched legs back as far as you can, you raise your vagina and thus enable your partner to enter you more easily

HAVING A SHORT PENIS is something that a man feels very ashamed of, and fortunes are made by companies that claim to be able to extend or enlarge the smaller man. The second posture is a very practical method of making intercourse possible for the man who is particularly underendowed, but I suspect that most women would find it too difficult or uncomfortable. In that event, the couple should consider alternatives to intercourse that will give satisfaction to both partners. These include masturbation, mutual masturbation, oral sex, and the use of sex aids.

CONCERNING PRAISEWORTHY MEN

According to Sheikh Nefzawi, a man "who deserves favors is, in the eyes of women, the one who is anxious to please them." As for the physical attributes of this praiseworthy man, when he is close to women "his member grows, gets strong, vigorous, and hard; he is not quick to discharge, and after the trembling caused by the emission of the sperm, he is soon stiff again. Such a man is relished and appreciated by women; this is because the woman loves the man only for the sake of coition. His member should, therefore, be of ample dimensions and length; he should know how to regulate his emission, and be ready as to erection; his member should reach to the end of the canal of the female, and completely fill it in all its parts."

THIRD POSTURE

This is an excellent posture to use when you want really deep penetration, and was perhaps inspired by the Yawning Position (see page 68) described in the Kama Sutra.

ALTHOUGH THIS POSTURE allows the maximum possible penetration, I recommend that it be attempted only when the woman is fully aroused, to ensure that her vagina is ready to be penetrated deeply. During sexual arousal, the vaginal canal undergoes a process called tenting, which involves the enlargement of its upper end to accommodate the deep-thrusting penis.

Leg positions
Kneel between her legs, then lift one of them onto your shoulder and put the other under your arm

Wait for full arousal
Because this position allows for maximum penetration, do not adopt it until you are fully aroused and your vagina is fully extended

FOURTH POSTURE

Varying the angle at which the man enters his partner can create a novel range of sensations for both of them. The Fourth Posture, in which the man places both his partner's legs over his shoulders before he enters her, enables a couple to find the most pleasurable angles of entry.

AN IGNORANT LOVER can unwittingly hurt both himself and his partner if he attempts to enter her at the wrong angle, but by raising her body a little before penetration he is unlikely to do harm. It is, of course, a good idea for him to have kissed, cuddled, fondled, and stroked her long before they begin sexual intercourse, so that she is properly aroused and her vaginal juices have begun to flow.

Straight legs
Keep your legs straight or, if you prefer, rest your calves on his shoulders

Angle of entry
Before penetration, lift her body slightly so that you can lower her vagina onto your penis at the most pleasurable angle

FIFTH POSTURE

◇

In this, the simplest side-by-side position, both partners lie with legs outstretched, and the woman raises her uppermost leg to allow the man to enter her. Nefzawi warns, however—with little or no justification—that the posture may cause rheumatism.

LOVEMAKING POSITIONS in which the man and woman lie side by side and facing each other, as they do in this one, are excellent for inspiring deep feelings of loving tenderness.

Deep penetration
Bend your leg and place it on his to ensure deep penetration

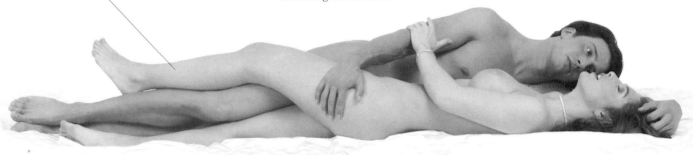

SIXTH POSTURE

◇

Because he enters the woman from a stable kneeling position, the man has his hands free to caress her back and breasts and stimulate her clitoris. Alternatively, he can hold her waist or hips and pull her back and forth on his member.

I THINK THIS CLASSIC rear-entry posture generates a powerful, primal eroticism. If at some time in our evolution we were truly ape-like, we would have copulated in this style. The buttocks are considered by anthropologists to give out strong sexual signals, and it has been suggested that the only reason the breasts in the human female are as fully developed as they are, compared to those of other primates, is because they are imitating the visual appeal of the buttocks.

Inviting posture
Part your legs and present your upturned vagina to your partner

Kneeling position
Support yourself on your elbows and knees

CONCERNING PRAISEWORTHY WOMEN

In describing the woman to be admired, Sheikh Nefzawi demands physical near-perfection, although to our eyes some of the characteristics he lists would be less than attractive.

"In order that a woman may be relished by men, she must have a perfect waist and must be plump and lusty. Her hair will be black, her forehead wide, she will have eyebrows of Ethiopian blackness, large black eyes, with the whites in them very limpid.

"With cheek of perfect oval, she will have an elegant nose and a graceful mouth; lips and tongue vermilion; her breath will be of pleasant odor, her throat long, her neck strong; her breasts must be full and firm; the lower part of the belly is to be large, the vulva projecting and fleshy, from the point where the hairs grow to the buttocks; the conduit must be narrow and not moist, soft to the touch, and emitting a strong heat and no bad smell.

"She must have the thighs and buttocks hard, the hips large and full, a waist of fine shape, hands and feet of striking elegance, plump arms, and well-developed shoulders. If one looks at a woman with those qualities in front, one is fascinated; if from behind, one dies with pleasure."

THE SEVENTH POSTURE

◇

The Perfumed Garden specifies that in this posture, the woman should be lying on her side while the man kneels and lifts one of her legs onto his shoulder, but it is marginally less difficult if she lies on her back.

WHETHER THE WOMAN lies on her side or on her back, this position is for acrobats and not to be taken seriously. You might, however, have a lot of fun incorporating it into a circus fantasy.

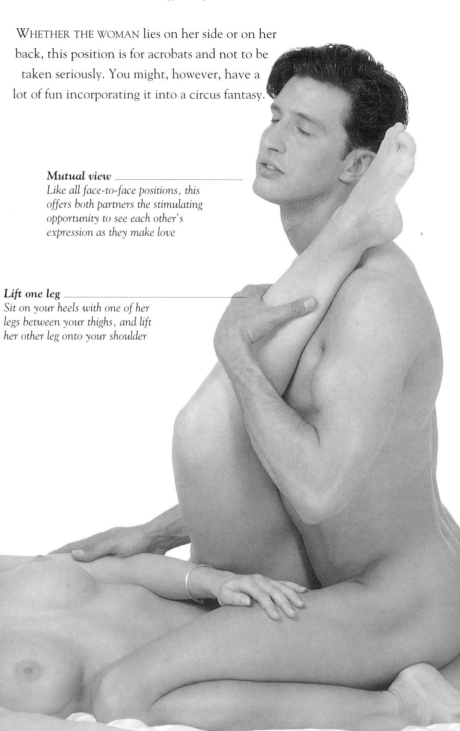

Mutual view ———————
Like all face-to-face positions, this offers both partners the stimulating opportunity to see each other's expression as they make love

Lift one leg ———————
Sit on your heels with one of her legs between your thighs, and lift her other leg onto your shoulder

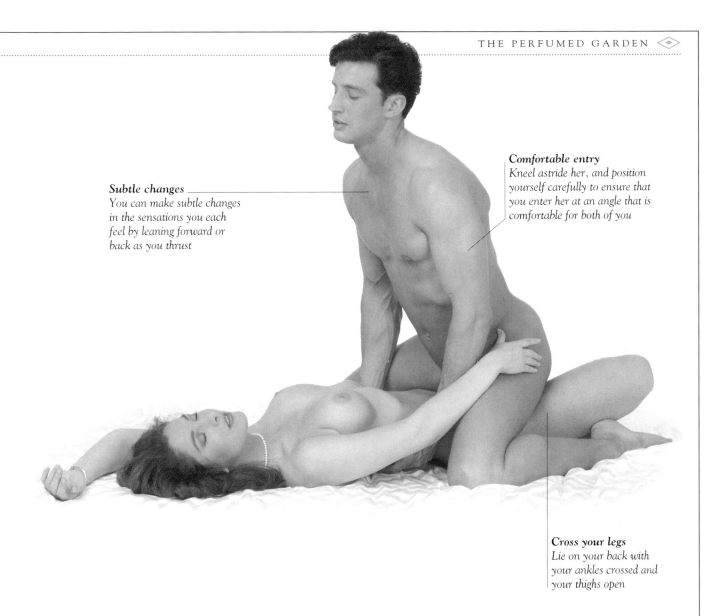

Subtle changes
You can make subtle changes
in the sensations you each
feel by leaning forward or
back as you thrust

Comfortable entry
Kneel astride her, and position
yourself carefully to ensure that
you enter her at an angle that is
comfortable for both of you

Cross your legs
Lie on your back with
your ankles crossed and
your thighs open

THE EIGHTH POSTURE

◇

By changing the position of the woman's hips, the man can vary the angle and depth of penetration, and because he is kneeling, his hands are free to caress her body. She can either pull her crossed legs back before he enters her or, as The Perfumed Garden suggests, cross her legs beneath her thighs so he can kneel astride her.

EACH OF THE TWO variations on this cross-legged posture has its own special advantages.
I suggest that you use the legs-pulled-back version when you wish for deep penetration and G-spot stimulation, and the legs-under-the-thighs version for clitoral stimulation.

THE NINTH POSTURE

This highly erotic posture can provide quite a variety of sensations because it has three main variants—two rear-entry and one face-to-face—and is one that lends itself to making love while clothed as well as when naked. In the rear-entry versions, the woman can either lie facedown across a bed with her knees on the floor, or stand and lean forward over it. In the face-to-face version, she lies on her back on a bed with her feet on the floor.

IN THE PRESENT century, this is the position that is featured most often in fantasies (and in the reality) of making love on the kitchen table, on an office desk, or on some other unconventional surface.

Easier thrusting
Keeping your body nearly upright and grasping her hips will make thrusting easier

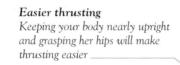

THE TENTH POSTURE

Grip the headboard
Reach back and grip the headboard or rail of the bed

Hip squeeze
Pass your legs over his hips and squeeze him tightly with them

Despite appearances, this is a position that puts the woman in charge—movement for both partners is limited, but she initiates it and he must respond to her rhythms. The woman lies on the bed with her legs stretched out and parted, and he kneels between her thighs. When he has inserted his member, the man bends forward and grips the headboard, and the lovers move back and forth with a seesaw motion.

PULLING AND PUSHING against the bed in this manner can improve the sensation of lovemaking so that it feels more decisive and exciting.

Kneel comfortably
For comfort, kneel on a pillow or cushion

THE ELEVENTH POSTURE

Although the woman's movements in response to her partner's are limited in this position, they are likely to be compensated for by the intense stimulation it provides and the depth of penetration that can be achieved.

THIS CLASSIC POSITION allows deep penetration and good clitoral stimulation. The movement of intercourse will pull the woman's labia rhythmically across her clitoris, creating a gentle, stimulating friction that may trigger orgasm.

Extra stimulation
Give him additional pleasure by stroking his buttocks and back

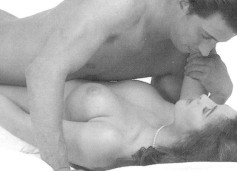

Soles together
After he has entered you, hook your legs over his and place the soles of your feet together

NAMING THE FEMALE PARTS

Drawing on the language of ordinary people, Sheikh Nefzawi waxes lyrical in praise of the female sexual organs. He identifies dozens of types, but gives special attention to what he calls simply "the vulva" (the Arabic word that he uses refers both to the vulva and the vagina). His description of this applies in particular to the sexual organs of a young woman:

"Such a vulva is very plump and round in every direction, with long lips, grand slit, the edges well divided and symmetrically rounded; it is soft, seductive, perfect throughout. It is the most pleasant and no doubt the best of all the different sorts. May God grant us the possession of such a vulva! Amen. It is warm, tight, and dry—so much so that one might expect to see fire burst from it. Its form is graceful, its odor pleasant; the whiteness of its outside sets off its carmine red middle. There is no imperfection about it."

As for the many variants described by *The Perfumed Garden*, their supposed qualities can often be discerned from their names alone—for example, the voluptuous, the crusher, the glutton, the beautiful, the hot one, and the delicious one.

Despite his humor, Nefzawi recognizes something most of us seem to have lost sight of today, and that is that just as all mouths and faces are different, so too are all genitalia. One thing that becomes clear about the Sheikh, on reading the elaborate details he gives in his descriptions of the different types of sexual nature of men and women, is how sexually experienced he himself must have been.

It's not just that he displays a grasp of sexual anatomy, both male and female, but also that he writes perceptively about the differences in human nature. In his description of the many different variants of male and female genitalia, he is really talking about the nature of the man or woman, rather than the style of his penis or her vulva.

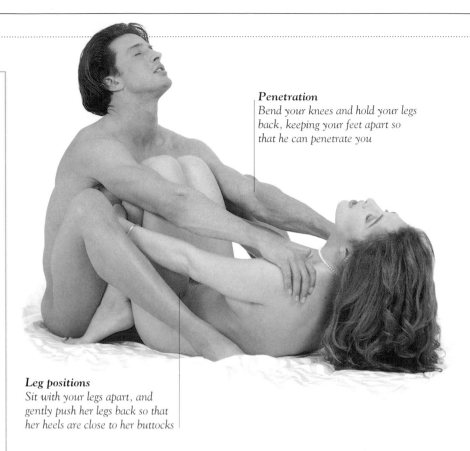

Penetration
Bend your knees and hold your legs back, keeping your feet apart so that he can penetrate you

Leg positions
Sit with your legs apart, and gently push her legs back so that her heels are close to her buttocks

FROG FASHION

Neither partner can move much in this position, in which the man is sitting and the woman is lying on her back, but it is both intimate and relaxed. At the moment of orgasm, Sheikh Nefzawi suggests, he should grasp her upper arms and draw her to him.

WOULD THE FROG PRINCE have used this, I wonder? Seriously, though, here is a position where he can use the leverage provided by grasping her shoulders, and she feels very contained with her legs tucked back. It's a curiously secure and cozy position.

Push gently
Keep your toes on the bed or floor and firmly but gently push her folded legs against her breasts

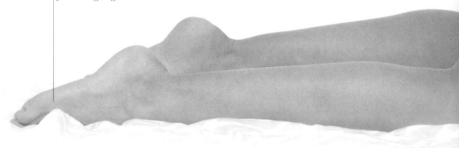

THE STOPPERAGE

*By pressing the walls of the vagina together and pushing the cervix forward, this position—
similar to the Pressed Position of the Kama Sutra (see page 79)—makes penetration
difficult, and once inserted, the penis presses on the cervix. There is a corresponding intensity
of sensation—so much so that Sheikh Nefzawi warns that the position is painful for the
woman. He suggests that it should be tried only by a man who has a short or soft member.*

IN HIS DESCRIPTION of this position and its effects, Sheikh Nefzawi demonstrates a
sound grasp of sexual anatomy. I think it is a good idea to heed his warning. Be very
careful when attempting this position.

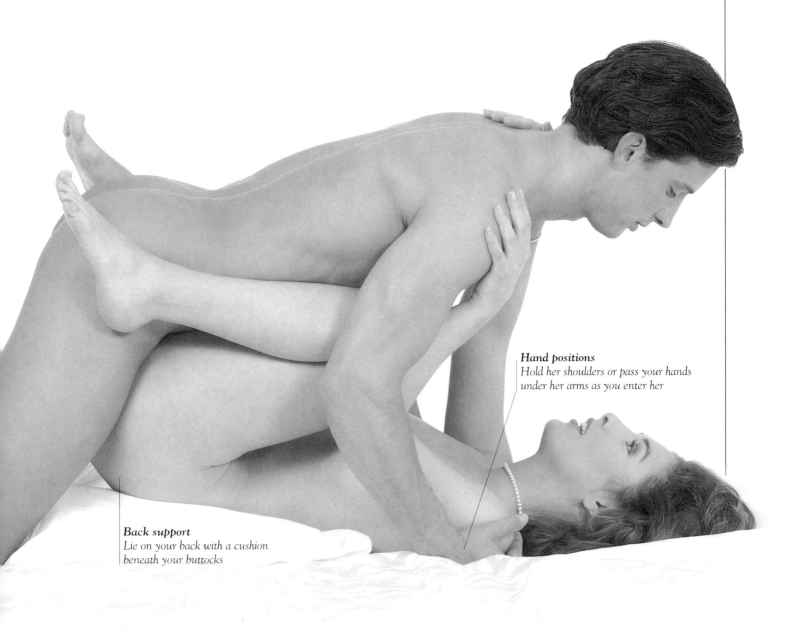

Hand positions
Hold her shoulders or pass your hands
under her arms as you enter her

Back support
Lie on your back with a cushion
beneath your buttocks

Hand holds
Put your hands
behind each
other's neck

Leg grip
Wrap your legs around
his waist and pull him
toward you

GRIPPING WITH THE TOES

The man is unable to thrust freely in this position, but it is good for expressing tenderness and as an interlude between more vigorous lovemaking. The woman lies on her back and the man enters her while kneeling between her thighs and bracing himself by gripping the bed or floor with his toes.

THIS IS ONE OF those positions in which the man can vary the angle of penetration by simply leaning either toward or away from his partner.

Lift her legs
Hold her legs close
together, lift them
straight up, and
rest them against
your chest

Thighs
Squeeze her thighs
with yours as you
gently enter her

WITH LEGS IN THE AIR

By squeezing her thighs together, the woman can increase the highly pleasurable pressure on her partner's member. As the tension between the vagina and the penis is great, the man should alternate light strokes with more forceful thrusts.

THIS IS ANOTHER excellent position for the older man who needs a lot of friction on his penis to stimulate him enough to climax. Because it does not provide much stimulation for the woman, however, other methods—such as oral sex or masturbation—should be used for her pleasure.

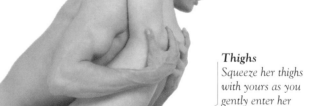

Raise her legs
Kneel at her feet, raise her
legs, and place them on
either side of your neck
before you enter her

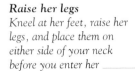

THE TAIL OF THE OSTRICH

◇

*The man can simply thrust, or he can vary the
sensations for himself and his partner as he does so by
raising or lowering her to change the depth and the
angle of penetration. If he does this, he should support
her with his hands under the small of her back.*

I THINK THIS POSITION smacks of male fantasy and
has little to do with making sexual intercourse
good for the woman. If she is happy to indulge her
partner in what almost amounts to a fetish (she is,
after all, almost upside down!), then all well and
good. But bear in mind that this could be very
tough on her spine and neck.

Upright posture
Only your head and
shoulders remain on the bed

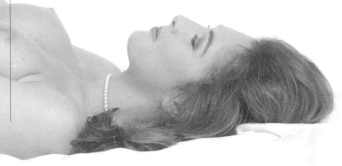

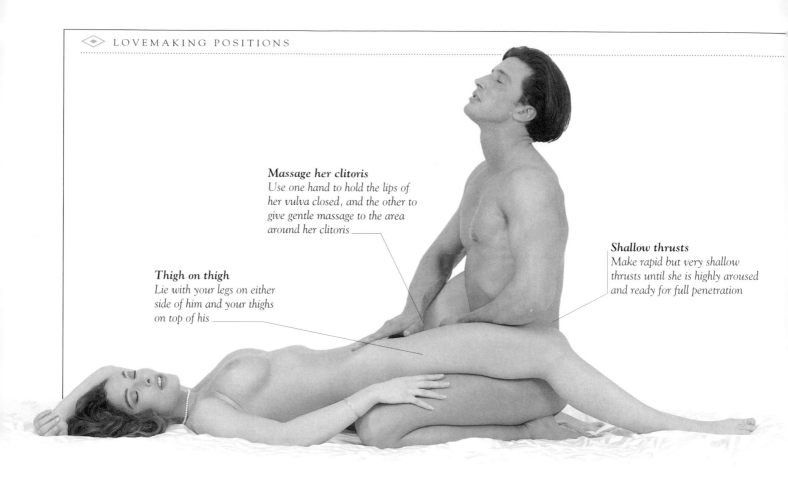

Massage her clitoris
Use one hand to hold the lips of
her vulva closed, and the other to
give gentle massage to the area
around her clitoris

Shallow thrusts
Make rapid but very shallow
thrusts until she is highly aroused
and ready for full penetration

Thigh on thigh
Lie with your legs on either
side of him and your thighs
on top of his

FITTING ON OF THE SOCK

◇

*More a type of foreplay than a true position, this aptly named gambit is
designed to arouse the woman for full penetration. While she lies on her
back, her partner sits between her legs and inserts the tip of his member into
her vulva, which he pulls gently closed around it with his thumb and first
finger. Moving his member gently back and forth, he rubs her outer lips
until his secretion moistens her vulva. He then enters her completely.*

THIS IS AN EXCELLENT method of using the penis as a dildo. Because
it's so different from intercourse and so locally focused on the inside of
her labia, including her clitoris, the woman may become extremely
aroused prior to penetration.

Views of the buttocks
When making love in this
position, you can see her
buttocks

INSPIRING AFFECTION IN A WOMAN

The Perfumed Garden stresses the importance of inspiring affection in the woman, and quotes the words of a woman on this matter:

"O you who question me, those things that develop the taste for coition are the toyings and touches which precede it, and then the close embrace at the moment of ejaculation! Believe me, the kisses, nibblings, and suction of the lips, the close embrace, the visits of the mouth to the nipples of the bosom, and the sipping of the fresh saliva, these are the things to render affection lasting. In acting thus, the two orgasms take place simultaneously, and enjoyment comes to the man and woman at the same moment."

RECIPROCAL SIGHT OF THE POSTERIORS

In addition to being relaxing for the man, this position allows him to delay his ejaculation because the sensations it generates are less intense than when he can thrust freely.

THIS CURIOUSLY IMPERSONAL method of intercourse allows each of the participants to fantasize about making love to someone other than their real partner. If they are in a long-term partnership where familiarity makes it difficult to feel desire, it could be very useful to foster such a fantasy. If, on the other hand, one of the partners showed a penchant for the position at an early stage of the relationship, I would be tempted to wonder who was rejecting whom.

Control the action
Sit astride him, insert his penis, then lean forward and move in whichever way gives you the most pleasure

Caress her back
Grip her with your thighs and use your hands to caress her back and buttocks

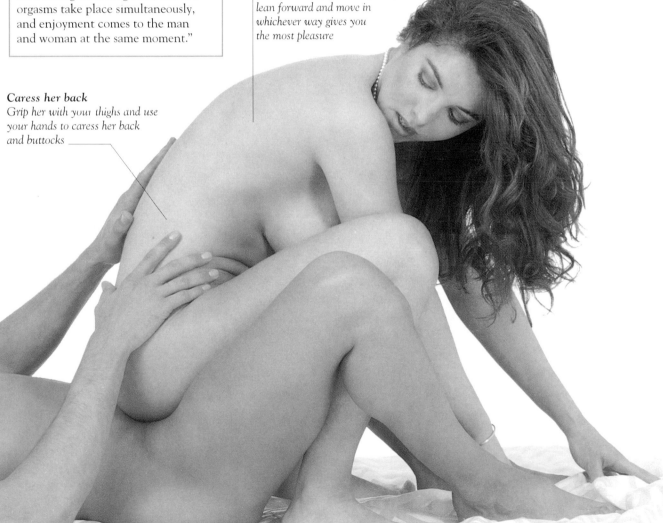

THE ALTERNATE
MOVEMENT OF PIERCING

In this unusual variation on the sitting position, the woman's role is an entirely passive one: after penetration, her partner moves her back and forth instead of thrusting from the pelvis. He can do this by alternately pulling her toward him and then letting her drop back slightly, or, as Sheikh Nefzawi suggests, she can sit on his feet and he can move them to carry her backward and forward.

THIS IS THE SORT OF unusual pose that is included in *The Perfumed Garden* as a thought provoker. The man would have to be such an athlete and yoga master, and his partner so very small, that it's hard to take such sexual advice seriously. Readers may be learning about the Sheikh's personal sexual fantasy—it certainly sounds like one of the unlikely stories that arrive daily in sackloads at the offices of many men's magazines.

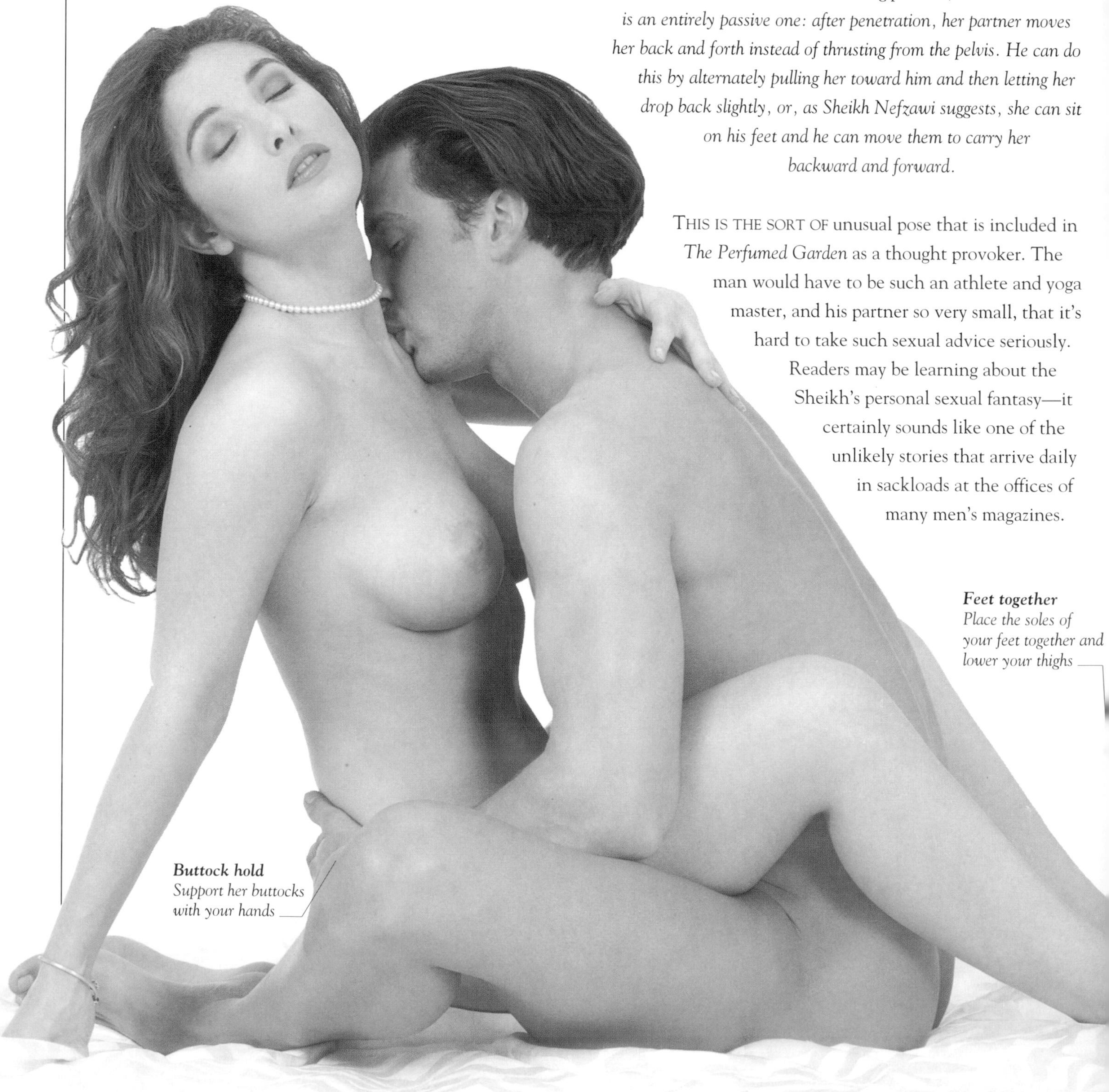

Feet together
Place the soles of
your feet together and
lower your thighs

Buttock hold
Support her buttocks
with your hands

THE MOVEMENTS OF LOVE

The author of *The Perfumed Garden* lists six movements for use during intercourse. The first three are the Bucket in the Well, the Mutual Shock, and the Approach.

THE BUCKET IN THE WELL
"The man and woman join in close embrace after the introduction. Then he gives a push and withdraws a little; the woman follows him with a push, and also retires. So they continue their alternate movement, keeping proper time. Placing foot against foot, and hand against hand, they keep up the motion of a bucket in a well."

THE MUTUAL SHOCK
"After the introduction, they each draw back, but without dislodging the member completely. Then they both push tightly together, and thus go on keeping time."

THE APPROACH
"The man moves as usual, and then stops. Then the woman, with the member in her receptacle, begins to move like the man, and then stops. And they continue this way until the ejaculation comes."

This is where The Perfumed Garden *comes into its own. Penetration can be an erotic and emotional experience in itself, and the idea that you can use special techniques to prolong or extend some of the heart-stopping excitement of such a moment is thrilling.*

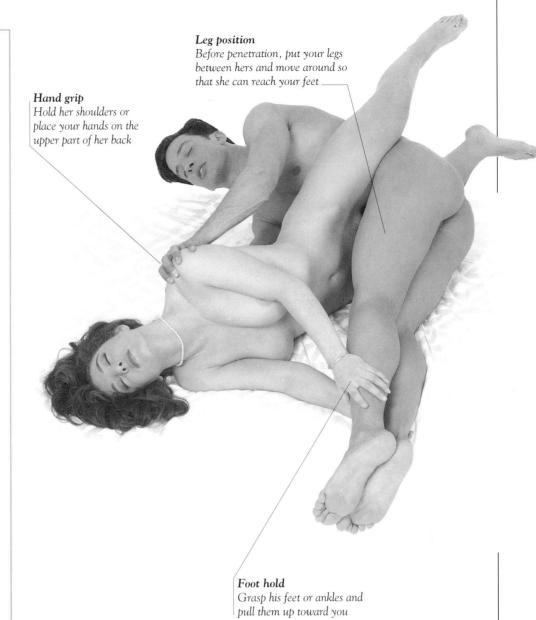

Hand grip
Hold her shoulders or place your hands on the upper part of her back

Leg position
Before penetration, put your legs between hers and move around so that she can reach your feet

Foot hold
Grasp his feet or ankles and pull them up toward you

THE RAINBOW ARCH

Although less relaxed than most side-by-side positions, this posture's unusual angle of entry provides novel sensations for the woman. Because of the shape that is formed by the entwined lovers, this position is also called Drawing the Bow.

I THINK THIS POSITION HAS more novelty than practical value, and it is not one that most couples would want to maintain for very long. But it's fun to try, and it can be incorporated into any varied lovemaking session.

POUNDING ON THE SPOT

This position will produce intensely pleasurable sensations for both partners. The man sits with his legs outstretched, then the woman sits astride and facing him and guides his member into her vagina.

FOR THE WOMAN, this lovemaking position bears similarities to horseback riding, because the movement of her thigh muscles is the same as that used in rising for the trot. The man's pleasure can be greatly enhanced if, every time she slides down onto his penis, she also tightens her vaginal muscles to grasp him strongly. This position has the added advantage of enabling the woman to be in control—their mutual pleasure is dependent on her choice of action, and it can make her feel powerful to have that choice.

Arms and legs
Put your arms around him and cross your legs behind his back

Rhythm control
Because you can move up and down freely, you can control the rhythm of lovemaking and the depth of penetration

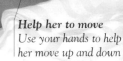

Help her to move
Use your hands to help her move up and down

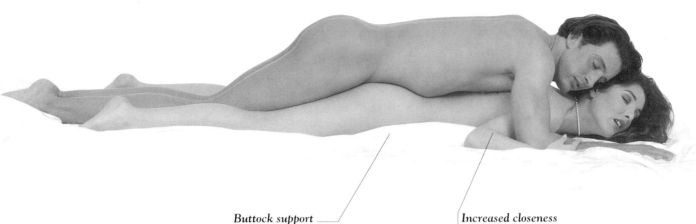

Buttock support
*Use a cushion or pillow
to raise your buttocks*

Increased closeness
*Entwine your arms around his to
increase the feeling of closeness*

COITUS FROM THE BACK

*As in other rear-entry positions, the man's member is aligned with his
partner's vagina in such a way as to ensure deep penetration, G-spot
stimulation, and a high level of arousal for both partners. This is, according
to Sheikh Nefzawi, the easiest of all lovemaking methods.*

THE USE OF A pillow or cushion to raise the woman's buttocks is a good
idea, because it presents her vagina to her lover at a more
accessible angle than if she were lying flat on her belly. This enables
the man to penetrate her deeply, and it also reduces the risk of his
penis accidentally slipping out of her vagina.

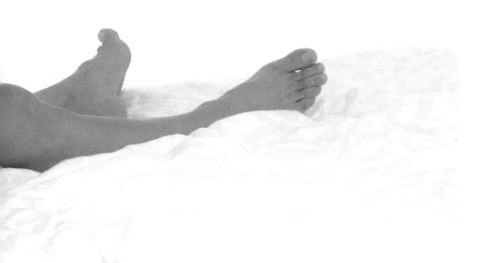

THE WOMANLY IDEAL

In addition to seeking an impossible
standard of female beauty, Sheikh
Nefzawi looked for compliance and
docility—in a word, subservience:
  "She speaks and laughs rarely, and
never without a reason. She never
leaves the house, even to see neigh-
bors of her acquaintance. She has no
women friends, gives her confidence
to nobody, and her husband is her
sole reliance. She takes nothing from
anyone, excepting from her husband
and her parents. If she sees relatives,
she does not meddle with their
affairs. She is not treacherous, and
has no faults to hide, nor bad reasons
to proffer. She does not try to entice
people.
  "If her husband shows his intention
of performing the conjugal rite, she is
agreeable to his desires and
occasionally even provokes them.
She does not laugh or rejoice when
she sees her husband moody or
sorrowful, but shares his troubles, and
wheedles him into good humor, till
he is quite content again.
  "She does not surrender herself to
anybody but her husband, even if
abstinence would kill her."

NAMING THE MALE PARTS

Just as Sheikh Nefzawi gave a long list of names for the vagina, so he does for the penis. Among the more inventive names he bestows are:
The Smith's Bellows—"The member is so called on account of its alternate swelling and subsiding again. If swollen up it stands erect, and if not it sinks down flaccid."
The Sleeper—"When it gets into erection, it lengthens out and stiffens itself to such an extent that one might think it would never go soft again. But when it has left the vulva, after having satisfied its passion, it goes to sleep."
The Impudent—"It has received this name because from the moment that it gets stiff and long it does not care for anybody, lifts impudently the clothing of its master by raising its head fiercely, and makes him ashamed while itself feels no shame. It acts in the same unabashed way with women, turning up their clothes and laying bare their thighs. Its master may blush at this conduct, but as to itself its stiffness and determination to plunge into the vulva only increase."

LOVE'S FUSION

Face-to-face, side-by-side positions such as this one permit the man to thrust vigorously and the woman to move with him if she chooses—Sheikh Nefzawi's instructions to the man conclude, "After having introduced your member you move as you please, and she responds to your action as she pleases."

THERE ARE NUMEROUS WAYS of intermingling legs in side-by-side positions, and many men and women are turned on by the sensation of their partner's legs entwining around their own. Just lying together, weaving patterns with the lower limbs, can be very arousing. Such positions are also conducive to relaxed lovemaking and are intimate in that they allow each partner to see the face of the other.

Leg over side
Hook your uppermost leg over his side

Leg over leg
Put your uppermost leg over her lowermost leg

Free hand
Use your free hand to caress her buttocks and to hold her close against you

Increased leverage
Press back with your uppermost leg to give you leverage when you thrust

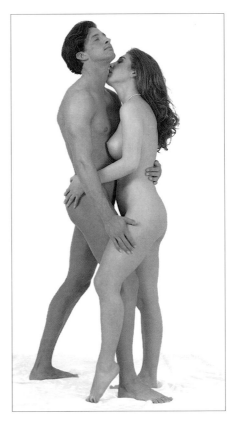

BELLY TO BELLY

◇

When a couple is making love in this first of his standing
positions, Sheikh Nefzawi recommends that they use the Bucket
in the Well technique of alternate thrusting (see page 125). This
can be used when both partners have both feet on the floor, as the
Sheikh suggests and is shown above, or when the woman hooks
one leg over her partner's thigh, as on the left.

THIS IS ONE OF THOSE downright lascivious positions that
celebrate lust and desire. Why bother to lie down when
you can do it so much quicker standing up? Why not
demonstrate the strength of your attraction by being direct?
Why not, just occasionally, enjoy the sheer recklessness of
intercourse without preliminaries when you desire each
other so much that you can't wait? There is a place in
everyone's sex life for such immediacy.

INTERCHANGE IN COITION

This is one of The Perfumed Garden's *woman-on-top positions, Sheikh Nefzawi's equivalent of the* Kama Sutra's *postures for "women acting the part of a man" (see page 86). For a variant of this posture, the Sheikh suggests that the woman kneel between her partner's thighs, with her feet on a cushion to put her at a suitable angle.*

THIS IS A SOPHISTICATED version of push-ups, where the woman's vagina and thighs are gripped tightly around the man's penis as she levers herself up and down. It is an excellent lovemaking position for the older man and his younger partner, because it gives the penis the extra stimulation that many older men need in order to climax. It also means that the active part is taken by the younger and, we assume, fitter partner. With subtle redirection of the angle of thrust, this position can be very good for the woman, because she can ensure that her clitoris is stimulated. The only snag is that she must be in great shape to get the best out of this position—it's a marvelous one for aerobics students.

> ❝ *No one is indifferent to the enjoyment that proceeds from the difference between the sexes.* ❞

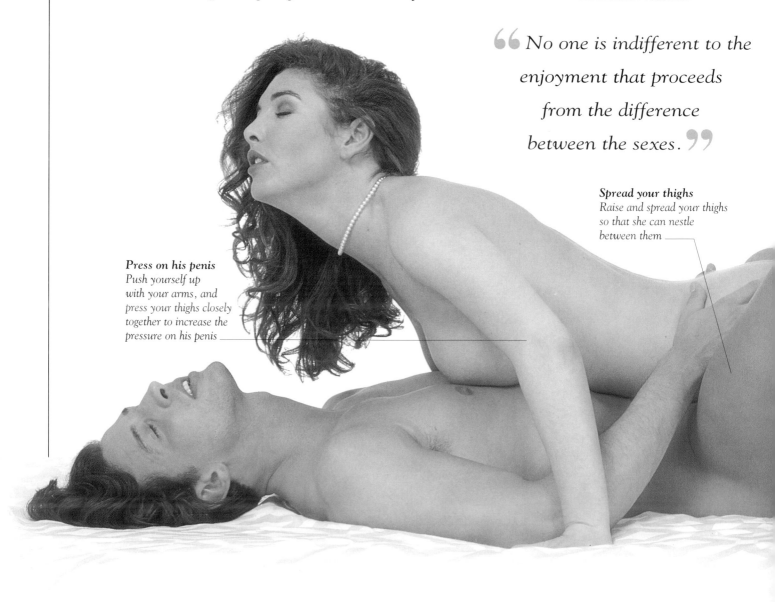

Press on his penis
Push yourself up with your arms, and press your thighs closely together to increase the pressure on his penis

Spread your thighs
Raise and spread your thighs so that she can nestle between them

DRIVING THE PEG HOME

◇

The second of Sheikh Nefzawi's standing postures is so named because the movement of the man's member is reminiscent of a peg being driven into a wall. If he is strong, the man can thrust satisfactorily while bearing the weight of his partner, but as his member is very vulnerable to damage in this position, great care should be taken.

THIS SEEMS TO ME to be such a difficult and risky sex position that perhaps it can be rated as a sexual activity alongside the Mile High Club: it's something so crazy you'd only really do it for kicks.

Hold on tightly
Wrap your legs around his waist, hold his shoulders, and keep your back straight against the wall

Raise your pelvis
Put a cushion or pillow under your legs to help raise your pelvis to a suitable height

THE STANDING POSITIONS OF LOVE

One of the difficulties with our modern world of sex therapy and marriage counseling is that we've acquired some very limited ideas of what constitutes good sex. Sexual politics filter into the bedroom, telling us, for example, that it's wrong to have sexual fantasies, especially those where we are being dominated by the opposite sex. If a sexual position doesn't do a lot for the woman, then we are encouraged to avoid it.

However, sex is not just about what happens within our bodies. Sex involves the use of the imagination, it is enormously variable, and the elements that make it diverse and therefore continually interesting and exciting stem from our emotional involvement in it.

The standing positions described in *The Perfumed Garden* and the other classic love texts bear witness to this. Most people associate lovemaking while standing with sudden passion, with the inability to wait a minute longer, with a kind of exhibitionism; above all, with the sort of excitement that overtakes you to the point of throwing caution to the winds.

And sometimes in sex, as in life, we want to act on our impulses instead of according to some kind of plan. Impulses are part of the fun of life, the element that makes it worth going on. This is what the various standing positions are all about.

THE RACE OF THE MEMBER

◆

In the basic version of this position, which was inspired by horseback riding, the man lies with a large cushion under his shoulders and draws his knees up. His thighs form a sort of V-shape into which the woman, facing him, lowers herself and from where she inserts his member into her vagina. For this more advanced version, he pulls his knees up toward his face and she sits astride his thighs to "ride" him.

FOR THE MAN who is curious to know what it feels like being a woman (and yes, there are quite a few), this is an interesting experimental position.

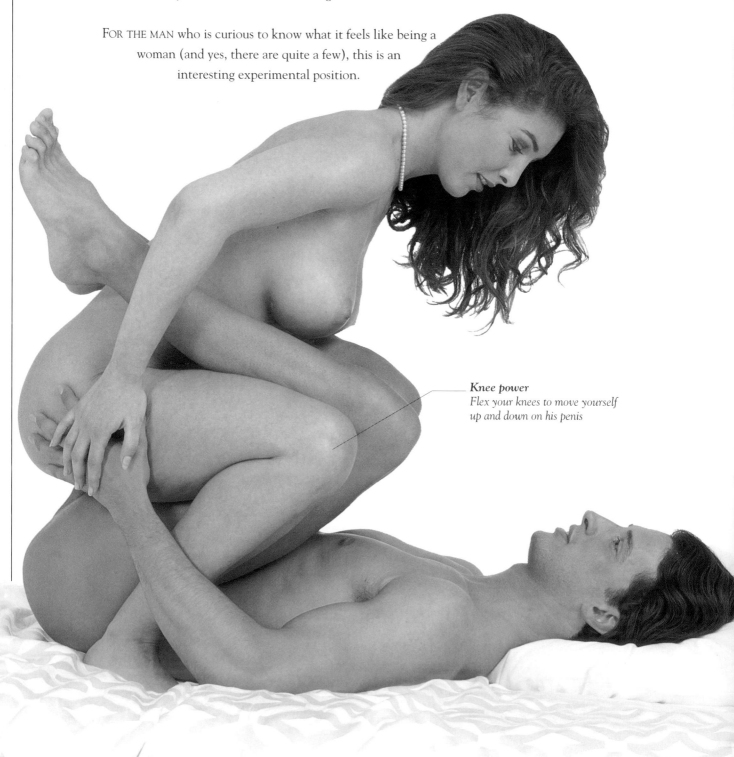

Knee power
Flex your knees to move yourself up and down on his penis

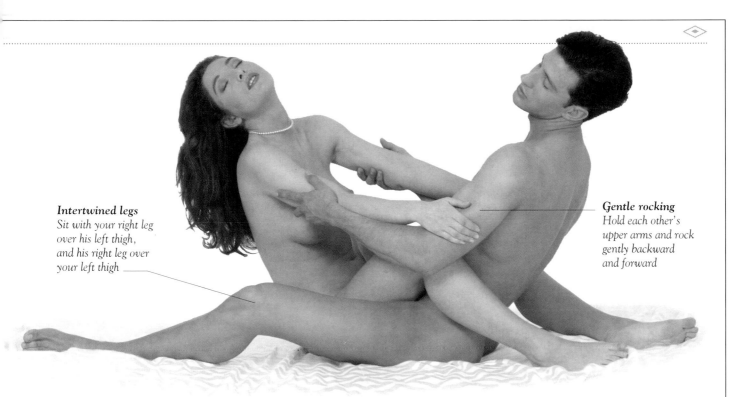

Intertwined legs
*Sit with your right leg
over his left thigh,
and his right leg over
your left thigh*

Gentle rocking
*Hold each other's
upper arms and rock
gently backward
and forward*

THE FITTER-IN

*A gentle rocking motion rather than a thrusting action provides
the stimulation in this unusual position. Gripping each other's
arms, the lovers seesaw gently backward and forward, being
careful to maintain a mutually enjoyable rhythm. Sheikh Nefzawi
(whose descriptions of intercourse usually assume that it is
taking place on the ground) recommends that the couple
maintain an exact rhythm "by the assistance of their heels,
which are resting on the ground."*

THIS FASCINATING POSE must be designed for the artists
among us, because the neatness of the interweaving of the
thighs appeals enormously to those who see everything in
terms of patterns. There's absolutely no reason why you
shouldn't enjoy sex in this way, taking pleasure in creating a
piece of living art composed of you and your partner.

FURTHER MOVEMENTS
OF LOVE

The second three movements recommended by Sheikh Nefzawi for use
during intercourse are Love's Tailor,
The Toothpick in the Vulva, and
The Encirclement of Love.

LOVE'S TAILOR
"The man, with his member being
only partially inserted, keeps up a
sort of quick friction with the part
that is in, and then suddenly plunges
his member in up to its root."

THE TOOTHPICK IN THE VULVA
"The man introduces his member
between the walls of the vulva, and
then drives it up and down, and right
and left. Only a man with a vigorous
member can do this."

THE ENCIRCLEMENT OF LOVE
"The man introduces his member
entirely into the vagina, so closely
that his hairs are completely mixed
up with the woman's. He must now
move forcibly, without withdrawing
his tool in the least."

THE ONE WHO STOPS AT HOME

The woman repeatedly raises her buttocks with a smooth, upward motion and then drops them again in a series of short, jerky movements. While she is doing this, her partner follows her movements, making sure that his member does not slip out and, as Sheikh Nefzawi instructs, sticking "like glue to her."

THIS TECHNIQUE IS probably effective only when used sparingly – intercourse consisting of nothing else but this would soon become less exciting and eventually extremely tiring.

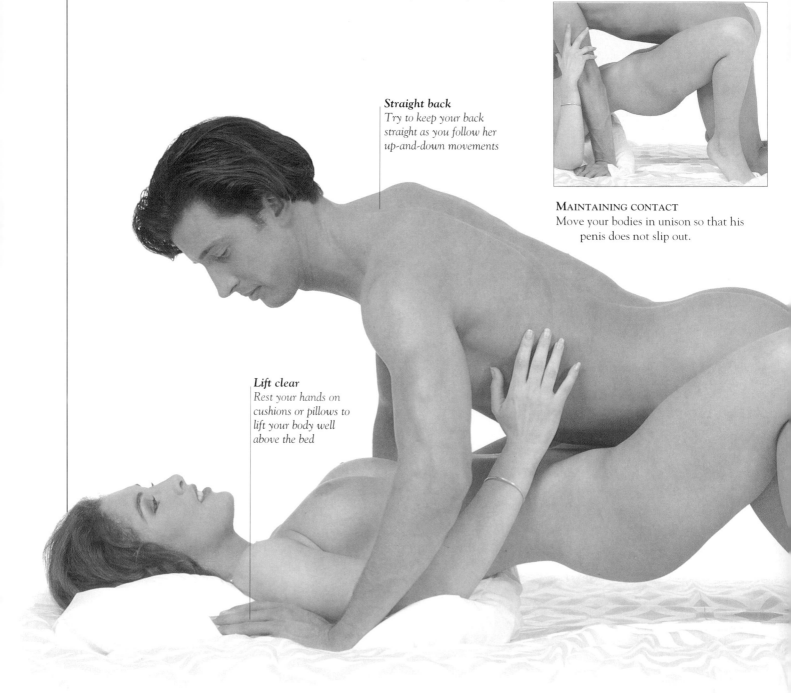

Straight back
Try to keep your back straight as you follow her up-and-down movements

MAINTAINING CONTACT
Move your bodies in unison so that his penis does not slip out.

Lift clear
Rest your hands on cushions or pillows to lift your body well above the bed

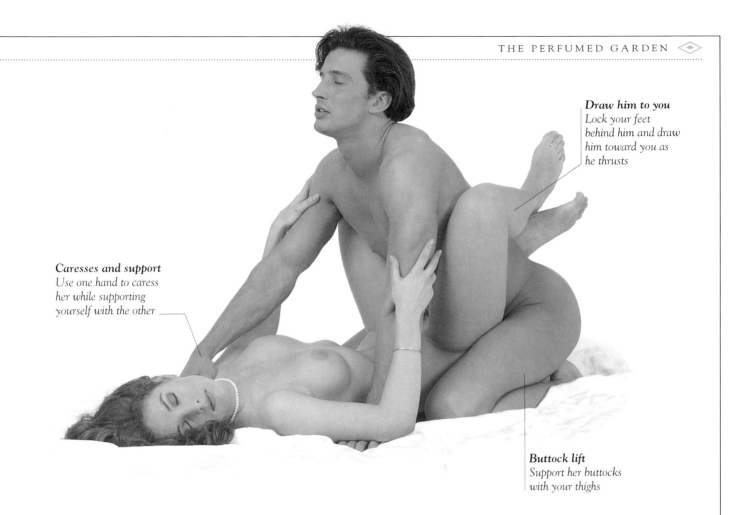

Draw him to you
Lock your feet
behind him and draw
him toward you as
he thrusts

Caresses and support
Use one hand to caress
her while supporting
yourself with the other

Buttock lift
Support her buttocks
with your thighs

THE SEDUCER

◇

*The seductiveness of a face-to-face posture combined with the pleasures of deep
penetration make this position enjoyable for both partners. There are two versions: in
the first, the woman puts her legs around her partner's waist, and in the second, which
provides even deeper penetration, she puts her legs over his shoulders.*

BY WRAPPING HER LEGS around his waist, the woman gives the man more leverage
as he thrusts. I always recommend that when lovers are adopting this position, it
should be the woman who guides the penis into her vagina. This gives her an
opportunity to knead and massage the penis before insertion,
providing her partner with some extra stimulation.

THE POSITIONS OF THE TAO

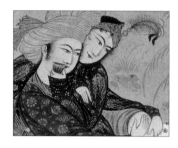

Taoism is an ancient system of religious and philosophical belief whose foremost proponent was Lao Tzu, who was born around 604 BC. Although its central text, the

Tao Te Ching, has traditionally been ascribed to Lao Tzu, scholars now date it to some two centuries after his time. At the heart of Taoism is the belief that ultimate harmony exists in the universe and can be attained by following the Tao. The word literally means "the path," but in Taoism it also signifies the functioning of the universe. To the Taoist, life is a balance of opposites in which everything that occurs has an equal and opposite reaction. Animating all that exists are twin forces: Yin, which is negative, passive, and nourishing, and Yang, which is positive, active, and consuming. The major component of woman's nature is seen as Yin, while a man is predominantly Yang. An imbalance exists between the sexes, so that woman needs the male force and man needs the female force. These forces are exchanged by sexual union, and it is at orgasm that they are at their most potent.

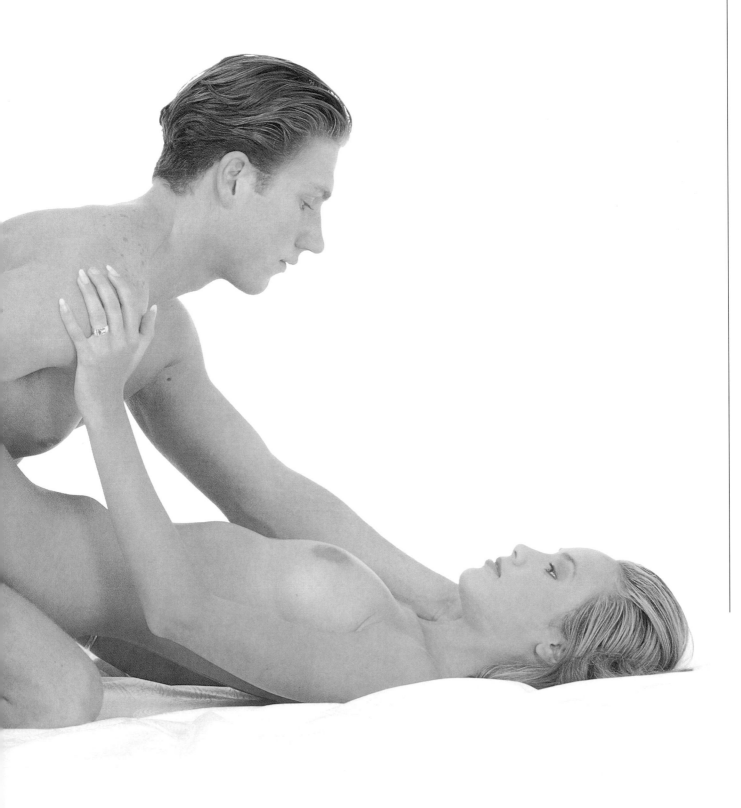

THE FOUR BASIC POSTURES

In the Taoist book *T'ung Hsüan Tzu*, the author, Li T'ung Hsüan, describes 26 positions for lovemaking, nearly all of which are variants of four basic postures. These basic postures are the Intimate Union (man-on-top); The Unicorn's Horn (woman-on-top); Close Attachment (side-by-side and face-to-face); and The Fish Sunning Itself (rear-entry).

THE DRAGON TURNS

This position is one that allows the maximum possible penetration, so the man should not attempt to enter his partner until she is fully aroused and her vagina has enlarged to its fullest extent.

THIS POSITION IS A pretty impersonal way for the male to find satisfaction. Eye contact is blocked by the woman's upright legs, the strain on her legs makes the whole experience uncomfortable for her, and the fact that her legs are held tightly together and upright ensures that her clitoris gets virtually no stimulation from his penis. I'd vote a distinct "no" on this one.

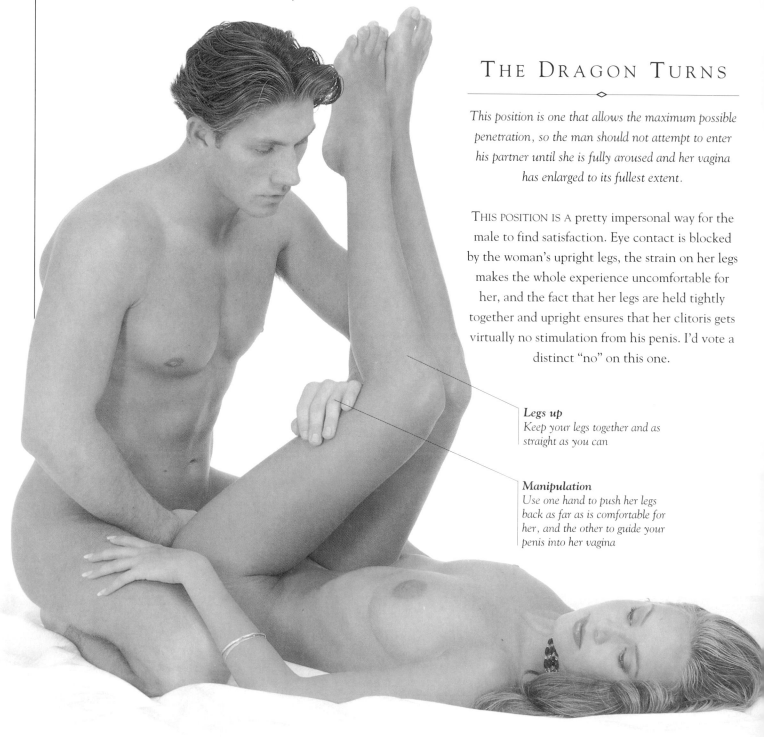

Legs up
Keep your legs together and as straight as you can

Manipulation
Use one hand to push her legs back as far as is comfortable for her, and the other to guide your penis into her vagina

A Silkworm Spinning a Cocoon

While lying on her back, the woman raises and spreads her thighs to expose her clitoris to powerful stimulation

ONE OF THE GREAT BENEFITS to the woman is that when holding her legs wide open she can imagine her vagina as a flower. Then, as she is stimulated, she can picture the flower opening, blossoming into orgasm. This kind of mental imagery helps many women reach climax.

Be responsive
Put your hands on his shoulders, cross your feet behind his back, and pull yourself up and down in response to his movements

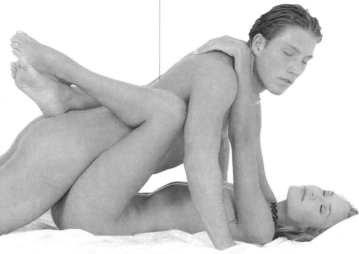

Change the tension
Use your free hand to lift her legs up onto yours, changing the tension between penis and vagina

Leg position
Keep your legs together and rest them on top of his

Two Fishes

Like a pair of spawning fish bending their tails around each other, the lovers lie side by side. After penetration, he lifts her legs onto his.

FOR SIDE-BY-SIDE intercourse to feel satisfactory, the man needs quite a long penis; otherwise, only a short part of it can remain comfortably inside her vagina, and it can easily slip out.

BUTTERFLIES IN FLIGHT

The man's movement is limited unless his partner is very light, but this position is useful when he is tired or when the woman wants to assume the male role and make love to him. Once the penis has been inserted, both partners stretch out their arms on either side of them, evoking the butterflies of the position's name.

THE TITLE OF THIS position is immensely evocative—the movement of the woman with her arms (wings) outstretched could, indeed, be undulating like that of a fluttering butterfly.

Push with your feet
Place your feet on his, and push against them to move yourself up and down on him

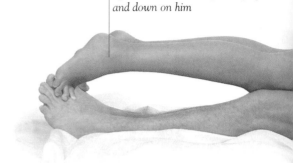

Free hand
Use your free hand to caress her

Knee position
Tuck your knees in behind hers

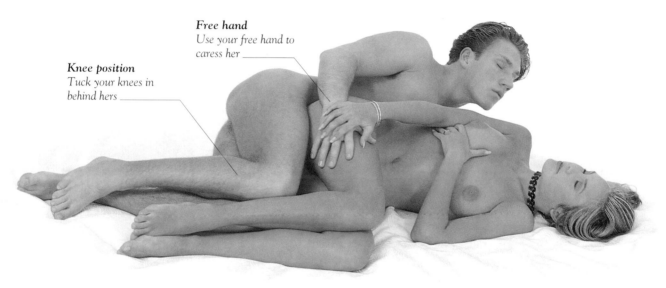

MANDARIN DUCKS

Its name inspired by the mating of mandarin ducks, this side-by-side, rear-entry position allows the man to thrust freely.

THERE IS SOMETHING SLY and seductive about slipping into your partner from the rear, especially if she has not been expecting it. For example, if she is asleep it can be a great way of waking her up.

Stretched legs
Both of you should stretch your legs out fully

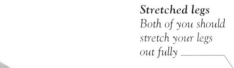

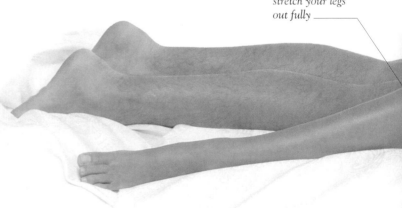

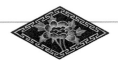

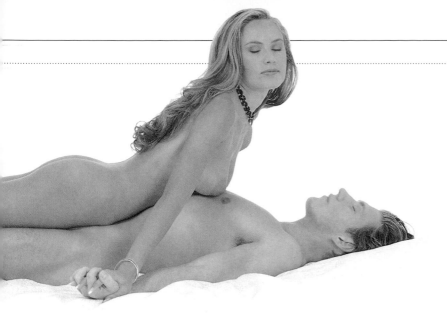

SWALLOWS IN LOVE

Another position with a name inspired by the courtship of birds, this gentle, man-on-top posture offers only moderate penetration but gives lovers an opportunity to express tenderness and mutual possession very eloquently.

THE PARADOX OF THIS position is that it is a method of feeling close to each other yet, through our stretched bodies, separate. This typifies the whole experience of intercourse: while intercourse may often create a feeling of mental fusion, the reality is that only the individual can experience his or her own sexuality.

Knee bend
Bend your legs at the knee before he enters you

Hold him
Grasp his waist with both hands

Forearm support
Take your weight on your elbows and forearms

THE PINE TREE

This position is ideal if the man's penis is short, because it provides deep penetration and, by using her entwined legs, the woman can pull herself up and down in rhythm with her partner's thrusts.

THIS IS A deep-penetration version of the good old missionary position, and the woman shows her enthusiasm for her man by wrapping herself around him.

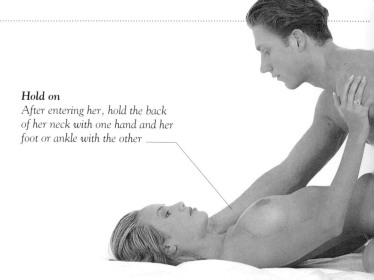

Hold on
After entering her, hold the back of her neck with one hand and her foot or ankle with the other

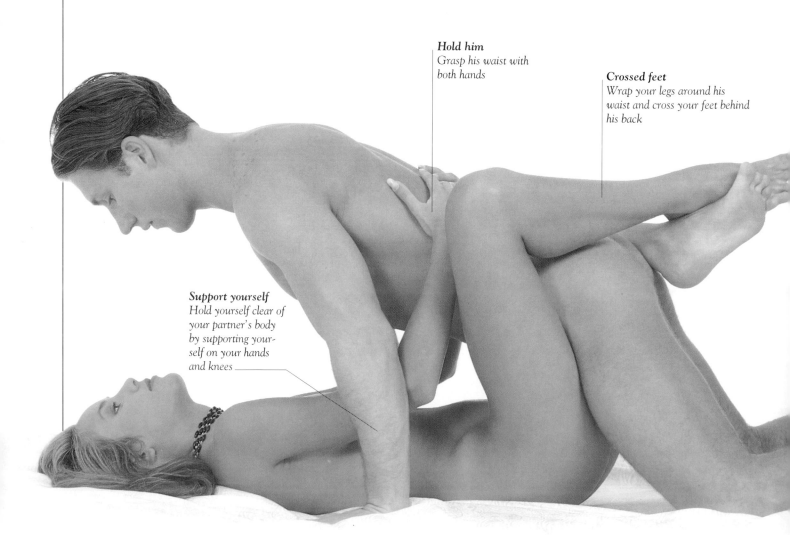

Hold him
Grasp his waist with both hands

Crossed feet
Wrap your legs around his waist and cross your feet behind his back

Support yourself
Hold yourself clear of your partner's body by supporting your-self on your hands and knees

THE GALLOPING HORSE

Feet in
Bend your knees and tuck your feet in next to his

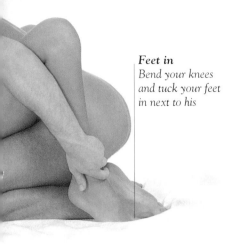

Like a bareback rider clinging to the mane and tail of a speeding horse, the man holds on to his partner's neck and foot, and so is able to thrust despite the restrictions of his kneeling position.

THE BEST WAY to make this complicated position work is to move up and down, but if the man is tall and the woman is small and light, forget it. It would either be impossible or positively dangerous should he fall over.

SEAGULLS ON THE WING

In most man-on-top positions, the penis thrusts downward in the vagina, but here, the penis and vagina are parallel, so that for both partners the sensations are somewhat different.

THERE'S SOMETHING ABANDONED about her slipping half off the bed and him thrusting wildly. But although his angle of thrust is interestingly different, his position means that her clitoris gets even less stimulation than usual. To help her get the most out of this posture, clitoral stimulation by his or her fingers would greatly add to the enjoyment.

Keep upright
Kneel between her legs, and keep your back straight to maintain the correct angle of penetration

Feet on the floor
Lie with your buttocks resting comfortably on the edge of the bed and your feet on the floor, if they will reach

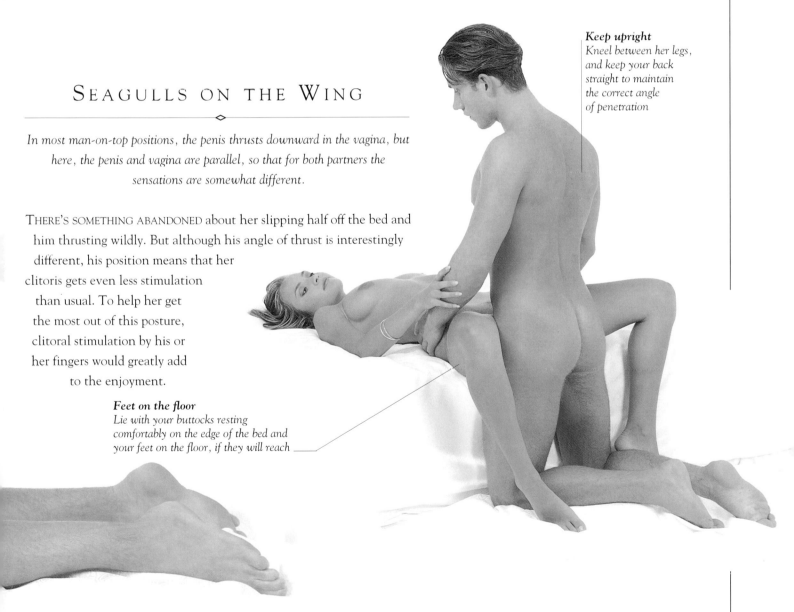

CICADA ON A BOUGH

Many couples find the relative anonymity of rear-entry positions exciting, from time to time, because they can fantasize more easily when they are not looking at each other. This position also provides intense stimulation to the front wall of the vagina and so to the highly sensitive G-spot.

IT'S HARDER TO GIVE EXTRA stimulation to the clitoris here, because the woman's genitals will be firmly lodged against either the pillow or the bed. This drawback can be overcome by using a vibrator, positioned so that every time her lover bears down on her, her genital area is pushed against it.

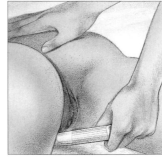

USING A VIBRATOR
To stimulate her clitoris, slip a vibrator between her pelvis and the pillow. Switch it on before penetration.

Toe hold
Grip the bed with your toes when you thrust

THE GOAT AND THE TREE

Although the man's movements are restricted, his hands are free to fondle his partner's face and breasts and stimulate her clitoris. This last possibility can prove useful because the woman is otherwise unlikely to reach orgasm in this position.

THIS DELIGHTFUL GAME could easily grow out of fooling around in casual circumstances. If she happened to sit on his knee during conversation; if she happened to kiss him as he was talking and he returned the kisses; and if one thing turned into another, before you know it, she could take him by surprise.

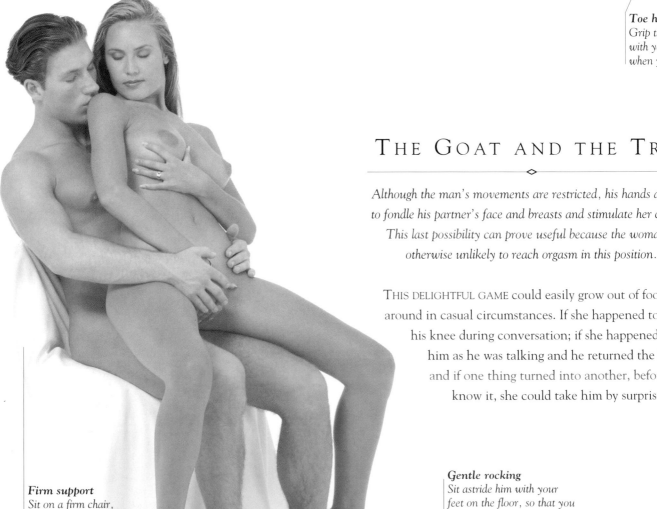

Firm support
Sit on a firm chair, preferably one with a supportive back

Gentle rocking
Sit astride him with your feet on the floor, so that you can rock gently backward and forward on his penis

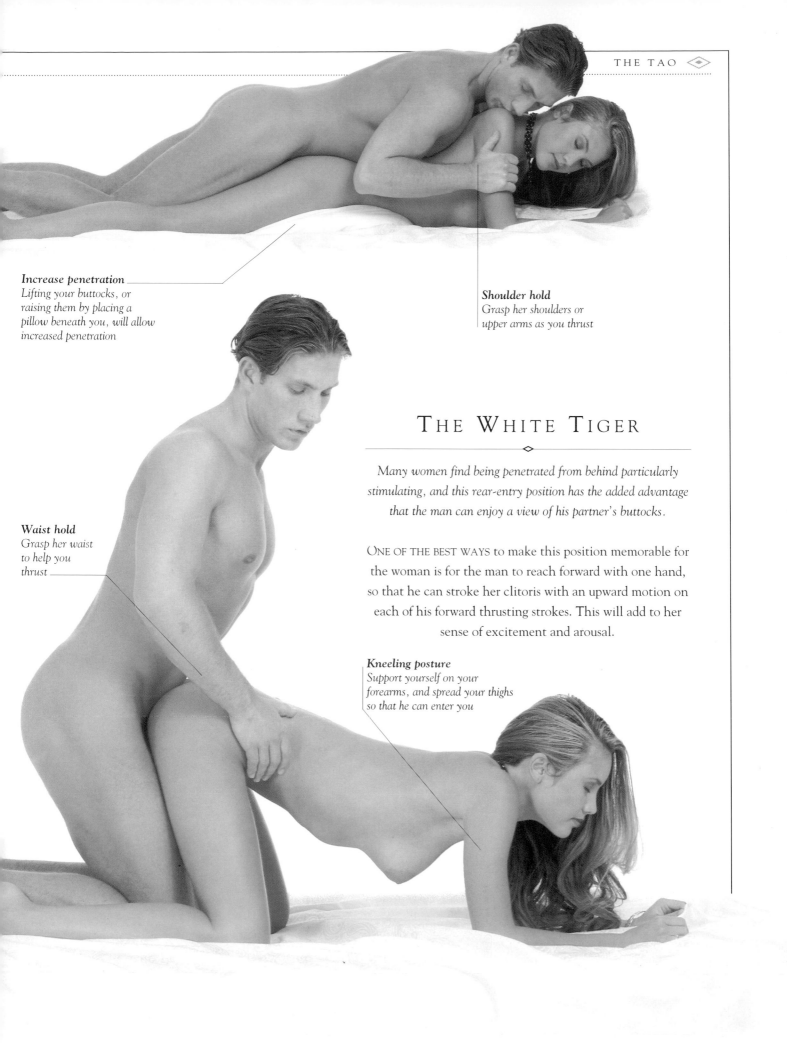

Increase penetration
*Lifting your buttocks, or
raising them by placing a
pillow beneath you, will allow
increased penetration*

Shoulder hold
*Grasp her shoulders or
upper arms as you thrust*

THE WHITE TIGER

*Many women find being penetrated from behind particularly
stimulating, and this rear-entry position has the added advantage
that the man can enjoy a view of his partner's buttocks.*

ONE OF THE BEST WAYS to make this position memorable for
the woman is for the man to reach forward with one hand,
so that he can stroke her clitoris with an upward motion on
each of his forward thrusting strokes. This will add to her
sense of excitement and arousal.

Waist hold
*Grasp her waist
to help you
thrust*

Kneeling posture
*Support yourself on your
forearms, and spread your thighs
so that he can enter you*

A PHOENIX PLAYING IN A RED CAVE

The vivid imagery of this posture's name hints at the deep penetration that it allows, but it may prove tiring for the woman if it is sustained for long. The man should wait until the woman is fully aroused before he attempts penetration.

THIS IS A WONDERFULLY evocative title for a position in which the woman lifts her legs to present the "red cave" for her lover's penis to "play" in. Because she is not able to move much, this is a position where the man should first use his penis as a dildo, rubbing it up and down her inner labia, then across or around her clitoris. On penetration, he might attempt some of the Movements of Love suggested by *The Perfumed Garden* (see pages 125 and 133).

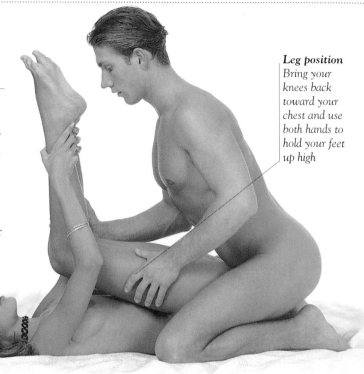

Leg position
Bring your knees back toward your chest and use both hands to hold your feet up high

A HUGE BIRD ABOVE A DARK SEA

This is another position that allows deep penetration. By lifting her legs, the woman changes the angle of entry of the penis so that, compared with the basic missionary position, stimulation is more intense for both partners.

BY PLACING HER LEGS over her partner's arms, the woman is both literally and figuratively making herself very vulnerable. Many women would feel emotionally unable to adopt this particular position unless they were deeply in love, so there is powerful meaning involved in it as well as profound physical sensation.

Gentle pressure
Lean gently forward against her thighs, without pushing too hard

Leg position
Raise your legs and pass them over his arms

Support her legs
Hold her waist and support her legs with your forearms

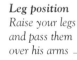

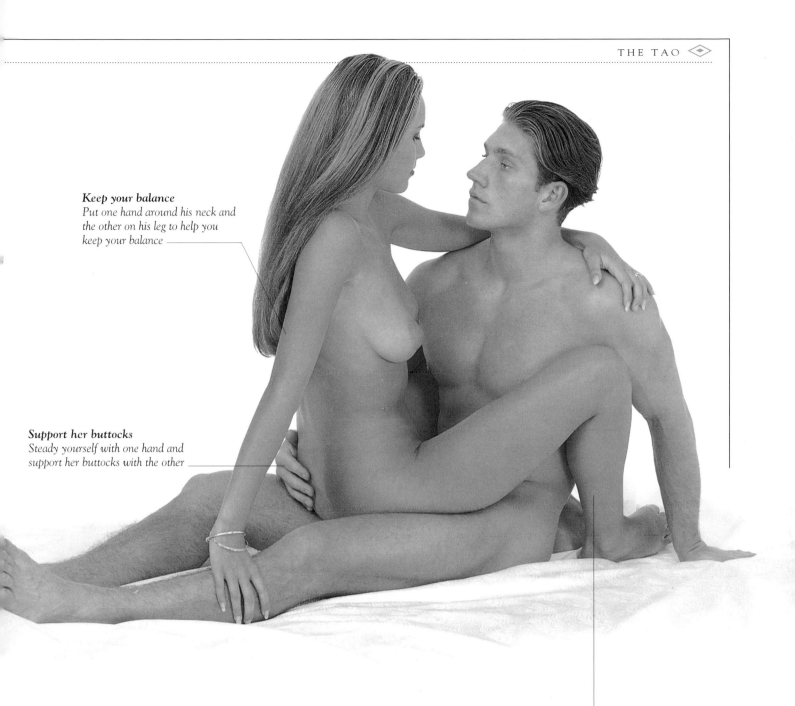

Keep your balance
Put one hand around his neck and the other on his leg to help you keep your balance

Support her buttocks
Steady yourself with one hand and support her buttocks with the other

Use your legs
Tense and relax your leg muscles to help you move back and forth on his penis

A SINGING MONKEY

◆

Neither partner enjoys much freedom of movement in this position—the man even less than the woman—but the couple can caress each other and look into each other's eyes, which can increase the feeling of closeness.

WHAT MAKES THIS DIFFERENT from similar woman-on-top positions is the placing of his hand under her buttocks; many women find this highly erotic, yet most men make little use of it. In addition to holding her buttocks, he can stretch them a little away from her perineum and anus, which can create very pleasurable sensations for her.

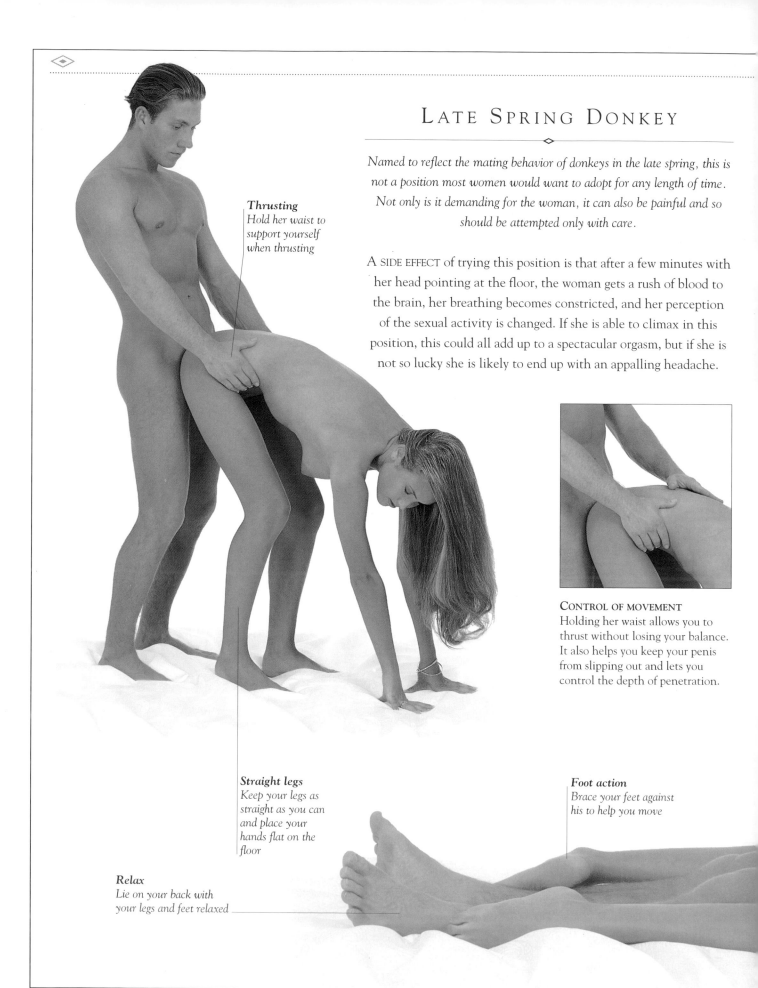

LATE SPRING DONKEY

Named to reflect the mating behavior of donkeys in the late spring, this is not a position most women would want to adopt for any length of time. Not only is it demanding for the woman, it can also be painful and so should be attempted only with care.

A SIDE EFFECT of trying this position is that after a few minutes with her head pointing at the floor, the woman gets a rush of blood to the brain, her breathing becomes constricted, and her perception of the sexual activity is changed. If she is able to climax in this position, this could all add up to a spectacular orgasm, but if she is not so lucky she is likely to end up with an appalling headache.

Thrusting
Hold her waist to support yourself when thrusting

CONTROL OF MOVEMENT
Holding her waist allows you to thrust without losing your balance. It also helps you keep your penis from slipping out and lets you control the depth of penetration.

Straight legs
Keep your legs as straight as you can and place your hands flat on the floor

Foot action
Brace your feet against his to help you move

Relax
Lie on your back with your legs and feet relaxed

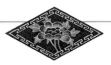

THE TAOIST PILLOW BOOKS

Over many centuries, probably from as early as 2,500 years ago, the wisdom of the Taoists concerning sexual practice was enshrined in "pillow books." Of these, the best known is the *T'ung Hsüan Tzu*, written by the seventh-century physician Li T'ung Hsüan.

Even today, the candid texts and beautiful but very explicit illustrations of the pillow books appear pornographic to some Western eyes. By contrast, to the Chinese who used them they were indispensable guides, not just to the mechanics of sex, but to living a long and full life in which uninhibited sexual expression played a central role.

Conversely, despite their candor and explicitness, the Taoist pillow books share some common ground with the less liberated aspects of the present age in excluding homosexual and lesbian practices. This exclusion was almost always justified on the philosophical basis that true sexual union is the interplay of equal and opposite forces as embodied in the two complementary sexes. Similarly, the books do not cover any form of sadomasochistic practice.

CAT AND MICE SHARING A HOLE

◇

Like other woman-on-top positions, this allows her to control the movements and rhythms of lovemaking. Although strenuous effort is usually required if either partner is to reach orgasm, this striving together can be mutually exciting.

I FIND THIS A disappointing position, considering the evocative title—my own version would include active stimulation by the hands and fingers. For example, he has both hands free, so he can caress any part of her body that he can reach, including her buttocks, breasts, and possibly her clitoris. She has little opportunity to give him any manual stimulation, unless she can support herself on one hand.

Keeping a rhythm
Push alternately against your hands and feet to move yourself backward and forward on your partner's penis

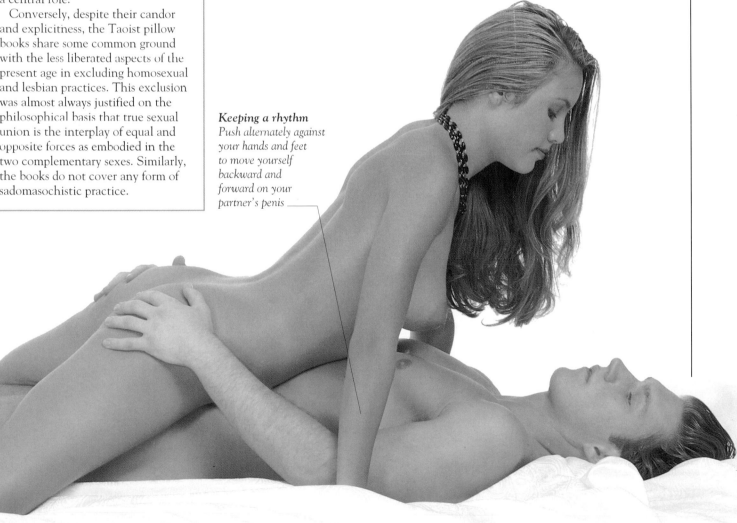

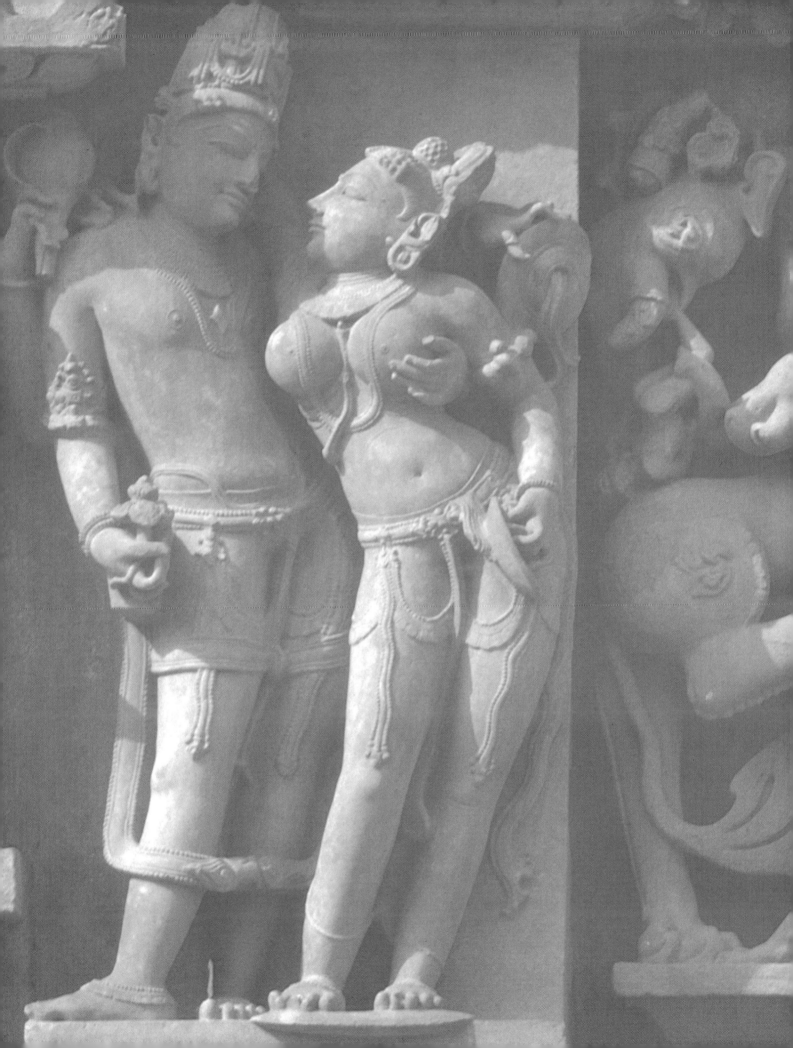

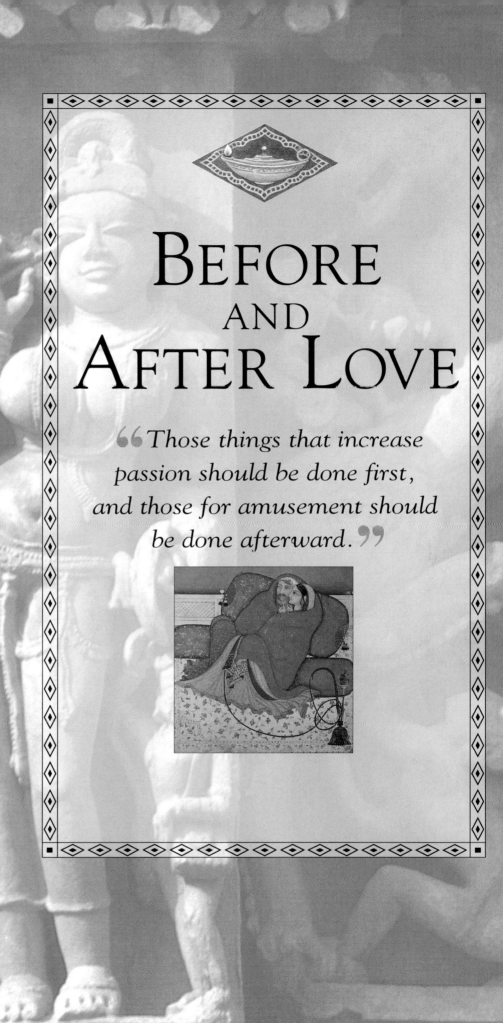

BEFORE AND AFTER LOVE

" *Those things that increase passion should be done first, and those for amusement should be done afterward.* **"**

SAFER SEX

Although sexual diseases were already in existence by the time the *Kama Sutra* was written, Vatsyayana makes no mention of them. People have always sought to avoid such infections, but the practice of "safer sex" is a very recent phenomenon. What has prompted this change in sexual behavior is the dramatic spread of AIDS (Acquired Immune Deficiency Syndrome). The term "safer sex" describes sexual activity that is unlikely to expose the participants to infection by HIV (the Human Immunodeficiency Virus), which is the cause of AIDS. The basis of safer sex is avoiding the exchange of bodily fluids (semen, vaginal secretions, and blood), because this exchange is the commonest way in which the virus is passed on. The most effective way of minimizing the risk of transmitting HIV infection during intercourse is to use a latex condom (*see page 154*) with a spermicide containing nonoxynol-9.

MINIMIZING RISK

When complete trust exists between partners, and each is confident enough of the other's sexual history to be reasonably sure that there is no risk of HIV infection, safer sex is irrelevant. But there is always the risk that any new partner will be infected. New partners should always practice safer sex. Blood tests for exposure to HIV can serve as an indicator that infection is unlikely.

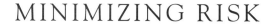

NON-PENETRATIVE SEX

◇

*As sensitive lovers know, penetration need not occur every time a couple has
sex. Dry kissing, embracing, stroking, and massage all express
closeness eloquently and with minimal risk of HIV infection. Mutual
masturbation may be used in the same way, but to be extra safe the active
partner should not allow any semen or vaginal fluid to come into contact
with her or his fingers or hands in case there are any cuts, abrasions,
or open sores on them.*

*Oral sex is a high-risk activity, particularly if the bodily fluids it produces are
swallowed. A degree of protection is provided by using a condom during
fellatio and a latex barrier ("dental dam") during cunnilingus, although
neither method is totally safe.*

*In accepting non-penetrative sexual activities as a valuable part of their
relationship, men and women who have any reason to suspect that they might
transmit the virus to each other will come to rely less on coital sex. When
intercourse does take place, they should always use a condom.*

HIV AND THE DEVELOPMENT OF AIDS

When HIV gets into the bloodstream, it attacks the immune system, the complex mechanism that enables the body to defend itself against disease. This damage eventually leaves the body vulnerable to other infections and liable to contract otherwise rare illnesses, including certain types of cancers and pneumonias. When a person with HIV begins to be affected by such illnesses, he or she is said to have developed AIDS. It is these illnesses, not HIV infection itself, that will eventually cause the death of a person with AIDS.

When a person is infected with HIV, the virus will be present in his or her blood. It will also be present in the semen of infected males and in the vaginal secretions of infected females. Anyone coming into intimate contact with these infected bodily fluids, as can happen during unprotected sexual intercourse, will be at high risk of contracting the virus themselves.

Once HIV has entered the blood, there is as yet no way of eradicating it, and AIDS will usually develop in about eight to ten years. You cannot, however, contract HIV from simple, everyday contact with someone who is infected. For example, you cannot catch it by shaking hands with them, or from their coughs and sneezes, or by touching objects they have used.

CONDOMS

The condom plays a central role in the practice of safer sex. Not only does it substantially reduce the risk of HIV infection, it also offers effective protection against other sexually transmitted diseases (and pregnancy). The main objections to the use of condoms are that putting them on interrupts the flow of lovemaking and that they reduce sensation for the man. The answer to the first problem is to get into the habit of making the task an erotic experience for both partners and an integral part of foreplay (*see below*). The second objection is to some extent valid, but in any case, some loss of sensation is surely a small price to pay for protection against HIV and other infections, including syphilis and herpes.

PUTTING ON A CONDOM

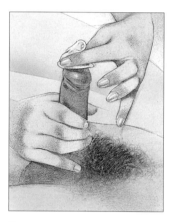

SQUEEZE OUT THE AIR
When you place the condom onto the end of his penis, squeeze it gently to ensure that it contains no air.

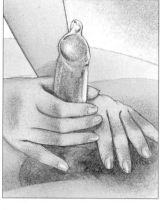

ROLL IT DOWN THE SHAFT
Use the other hand to roll the condom down the shaft of his penis to the base, using a slow and even action.

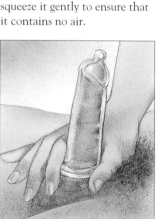

WITHDRAWAL
Remind him to hold the condom on his penis after ejaculation and to withdraw before his erection subsides.

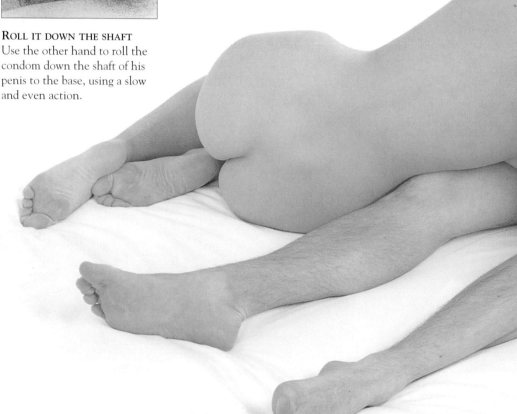

USING A CONDOM

Make slipping a condom onto your lover's penis a loving, sensual, and erotic action, and turn it into an integral part of your lovemaking. Begin by giving him a delicate genital massage, and then change your hand action from massage to gentle masturbation.

REMOVE THE CONDOM carefully from its packet, squeeze out the air by holding the tip between thumb and forefinger (a trapped air bubble could cause it to split during intercourse), and use slow, sensuous movements to roll it into place. If your partner is not circumcised, gently push back his foreskin before unrolling the condom.

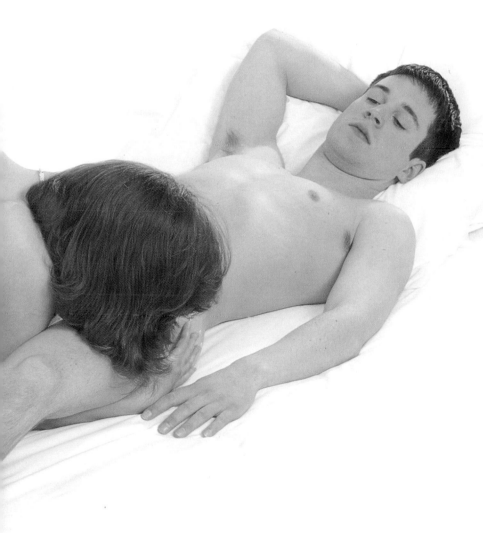

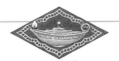

CHOOSING AND USING YOUR CONDOMS

Condoms must be of dependable quality—for maximum safety, avoid obscure brands and fancy (especially bumpy) patterns, and check the use-by date. Just as importantly, a condom must be used correctly, because if it is not tight it might slip off the penis or leak semen into the vagina during intercourse.

Condoms must never be reused, and you should be careful to avoid bringing them into contact with oil-based products such as massage oils and creams, baby oil, and petroleum jelly (including Vaseline). Condoms are made of latex, and this material is damaged and weakened by contact with oil. If you need to use a lubricant, choose a water-based product such as K-Y Jelly.

Some men and women dislike using condoms, but this is a learned aversion that can be unlearned relatively easily. As an alternative, try using female condoms, which fit into the vagina rather than over the penis. For protection against infection during oral sex, use oral shields ("dental dams") for cunnilingus and condoms for fellatio; flavored condoms can make fellatio through a condom more enjoyable for a woman.

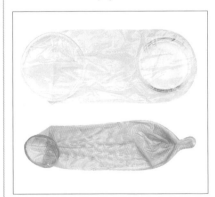

MALE AND FEMALE CONDOMS
The female condom (top), which is relatively new on the market, fits inside the vagina. The male condom (bottom) fits over the penis.

PROLONGING THE MOOD

Partners who genuinely care for each other will want to prolong the unique closeness that lovemaking brings, by staying close emotionally and physically. Having just reaffirmed a continuing intimate bond, some couples find that after making love they can talk more easily about things that matter to them either as a couple or as individuals. It is important to

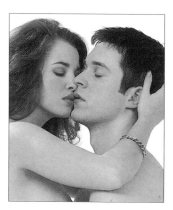

be able to communicate about what you enjoy most about your sexual relationship, and indeed to feel free to tell your partner if there is anything about your lovemaking that you would like to change. Some couples talk about these things while making love, while others find it easier afterward, as they look back on the pleasures, and the occasional disappointments, they have shared. Often, though, a couple will want to resume their lovemaking, in which case it might be

necessary for the woman to masturbate the man to get him erect again. If they do not intend to make love again, but the woman was not able to reach a satisfactory climax, the considerate thing for the man to do would be to masturbate his partner to help her achieve orgasm.

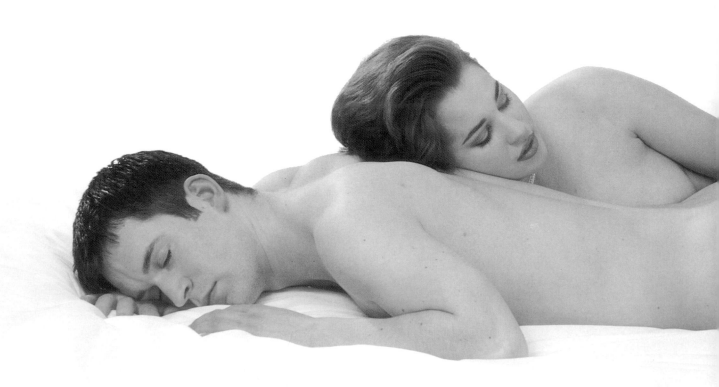

WHAT TO DO AFTERWARD

The *Kama Sutra*, mindful that lovers wish to prolong the special mood of intimacy that lovemaking creates between them, advises them on the sensual delights they should share immediately afterward. The details have, inevitably, changed a lot over the centuries, but the principles behind Vatsyayana's main recommendations still make sense:

"At the end of the congress, the lovers with modesty, and not looking at each other, should go separately to the washing room. After this, sitting in their own places, they should eat some betel leaves, and the citizen should apply with his own hand to the body of the woman some pure sandalwood ointment, or ointment of some other kind.

"He should then embrace her with his left arm, and with agreeable words should cause her to drink from a cup held in his own hand, or he may give her water to drink. They can eat sweetmeats, or anything else, according to their likings, and may drink fresh juice, soup, gruel, extracts of meat, sherbet, the juice of mango fruits, the extract of the juice of the citron tree mixed with sugar, or anything that may be liked in different countries, and known to be sweet, soft, and pure."

REKINDLING THE EXCITEMENT

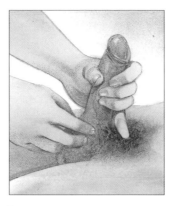

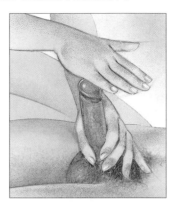

RENEWING AN ERECTION
Gently fondle his testicles with one hand while sliding the other up and down his penis.

ENHANCING AROUSAL
Brush the head of his penis by making featherlight, circular strokes with your palm.

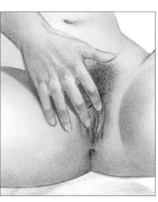

HELPING HER TO ORGASM
If your partner has not been able to reach a climax during intercourse, or if she wants more orgasms but you are not yet ready to make love again, help her by using your fingers to stimulate her clitoris. Gently run your fingertips along the underside, on each side, and on top of it.

SUSTAINING THE HARMONY

Most lovers do not want to dissipate the warm glow of lovemaking by simply turning over and going to sleep, or by doing anything that is either physically or intellectually demanding. Some simply like to lie quietly in each other's arms, while others prefer to follow love with a gentle, but not too sensual, massage. If they choose to get up, they may want to sustain the relaxed, harmonious mood by eating together, or enjoying an undemanding activity such as listening to music or taking a leisurely walk.

INDEX

ADDITIONAL READING

ANAND, MARGO
The Art of Sexual Ecstasy
Jeremy P. Tarcher, Inc., Los Angeles, 1991

BROUGH, JOHN
Poems from the Sanskrit
Viking Penguin, New York, 1977

BURTON, SIR RICHARD
AND ARBUTHNOT,
FORSTER FITZGERALD
The Illustrated Kama Sutra, Ananga-Ranga, and Perfumed Garden: The Classic Eastern Love Texts
Inner Traditions International, Ltd.,
Rochester, VT, 1991

BURTON, SIR RICHARD
AND ARBUTHNOT,
FORSTER FITZGERALD
The Kama Sutra of Vatsyayana
Berkley Publishing Group, New York, 1984

BURTON, SIR RICHARD
AND ARBUTHNOT,
FORSTER FITZGERALD
The Perfumed Garden of the Shaykh Nefzawi
Lightyear Press, Inc., Laurel, NY, 1992

CAUTHERY, DR. PHILIP,
STANWAY, DR. ANDREW, AND
COOPER, FAYE
The Complete Guide to Sexual Fulfillment
Prometheus Books, Buffalo, NY, 1986

CHANG, JOLAN,
The Tao of Love and Sex
Viking Penguin, New York, 1991

COMFORT, ALEX
The Joy of Sex
Simon & Schuster, New York, 1974

COMFORT, ALEX
More Joy of Sex
Pocket Books, New York, 1991

HOFER, JACK
The Joy of Sensual Massage
The Putnam Publishing Group,
New York, 1989

HOOPER, ANNE
Anne Hooper's Pocket Sex Guide
Dorling Kindersley, New York, 1994

HOOPER, ANNE
The Ultimate Sex Book
Dorling Kindersley, New York, 1992

ISHIHARA, AKIRA AND
LEVY, HOWARD
The Tao of Sex
Integral Publishing, Lower Lake, CA, 1989

JANUS, SAMUEL S. AND
JANUS, CYNTHIA L.
The Janus Report on Sexual Behavior
John Wiley & Sons, Inc., New York, 1993

LACROIX, NITYA
Sensual Massage
Henry Holt & Company, New York, 1990

REINISCH, JUNE M. AND
BEASLEY, RUTH
The Kinsey Institute New Report on Sex
St. Martin's Press, Inc., New York, 1990

STOPPARD, DR. MIRIAM
The Magic of Sex
Dorling Kindersley, New York, 1992

ACKNOWLEDGMENTS

Studio photography:
Jules Selmes, assisted by Steve Head.
Bath supplied by The Water Monopoly

Hair and make-up:
Jill Hornby, Karen Fundell,
and Melissa Lackersteen

Illustrators:
Jane Craddock-Watson and
John Geary

Picture research:
Diana Morris

Production consultant:
Lorraine Baird

Picture credits:
Chester Beatty Dublin/Bridgeman
Art Library 25;
E. T. Archive: 16, 151;
Lownes Collection/Bridgeman
Art Library: 11 bottom, 15, 65;
Private Collection/Bridgeman
Art Library: 6, 7, 8, 66, 90;
Victoria and Albert
Museum/Bridgeman Art
Library: 9 top, 10, 11 top,
22, 45, 136.
The Charles Walker
Collection: 1, 2-3, 9, 14-15,
24-25, 44-45, 64-65,
150-151;

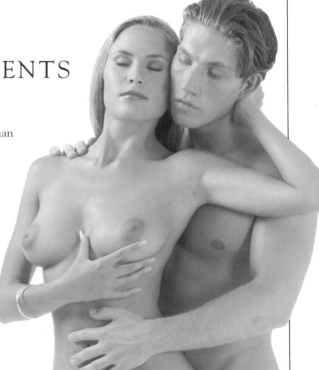